SNEEZING SEASONS

(The inside story about allergies
and immunology
told by Henry, an antibody)

by

Gail M. Galvan

SNEEZING SEASONS

by

Gail M. Galvan

EDITED BY (1986 Version): Sharon Radetsky-Hampal

ILLUSTRATIONS by: Michael Rasmussen (For scanning purposes, it was necessary to trace over artist's work)

COVER DESIGN by: Tony and Gail Galvan

Published by:

INFI∞ITY
PUBLISHING.COM
519 West Lancaster Avenue
Haverford, PA 19041-1413
ORDER BOOK FROM: buybooksontheweb.com

ISBN: 0-7414-0019-7

Printed in the United States of America

AUTHOR'S NOTE

"For those who sneeze, wheeze, itch, swell up and feel miserable at times, I want you to know you are not alone. There are many millions who share similar agony and frustration. Though your common affliction may invade your life, alter your temperament, and turn your body into a battlefield, immunological equilibrium is still within your grasp.

Just believe that each day, every moment that you fight against sickness and work conscientiously toward wellness, makes a difference. Setbacks will come, but the bad days and moments will disappear as the clouds part ways. LOOK FOR THE RAINBOW AFTER THE RAINFALL. FOLLOW THE SUN AND YOU WILL BE OKAY. GOOD LUCK FROM HENRY AND THE REST OF US."

Gail Galvan & Henry!

Gail M. Galvan, L.P.N.
B.A. Health and Wellness Education

DEDICATION

Dedicated to the creative and healthful spirit that lives within us all and of course to mom and dad, with love.

ACKNOWLEDGMENTS

I wish to express my sincere appreciation to several people who offered guidance, encouragement, and assistance in preparation of the manuscript: To Sharon for her editorial advice and genuine insight regarding the allergy/asthma problem, to Dr. William E. Rhodes, for his warm heart, creative energy and philosophical wisdom, to Anne Hatcher, R.D., Ed.D., for her support and nutritional expertise and to Mr. Roy Raney from the currently named National Jewish Research and Medical Center for his important insight after reviewing an early draft.

Thanks also to Mr. Michael Rasmussen for bringing the characters, Henry and George, to life. I'm grateful to Joan M. Kolodziej, for her word processing skills and extra effort and to Vivian at Nerdworld, "Fabulous job!"

A final draft is the accumulation of an original idea which connected with a wide variety of serendipitous and purposeful chain of events throughout its entire development. Thank you all for helping build the fragmented parts of Sneezing Seasons and making the book whole.

Special credit and thanks also to author Dr. Ronald J. Glasser, for his book, *The Body Is The Hero*, 1976, 1979, a Bantam Book published by arrangement with Random House, Inc. Anything medically incorrect, go ahead and blame "Henry".

A late entry, 1999 grateful acknowledgment goes out to Buy Books in Bryn, Mawr, Pennsylvania. One of my literary dreams, this book, lives because of you and the pioneering service Buy Books has created and offers to unknown, as well as already established, writers.

CONTENTS

CHAPTER 1

There's a war going on inside hypersensitive bodies between the antigens and us, the antibodies. Battlegrounds within bloodstreams, leaky fluids, cells, and body organs, a conglomeration of chemical reactions occur every minute. Sometimes we win, sometimes we lose, but my comrades and I always give it a good fight.

My name is Henry. I'm an antibody, a specialist in hypersensitivity. My enemies call me a scout, someone to be wary of and avoid at all costs. You can think of me as an agent, a good guy or a bad guy, because I can be both, as some of the following stories will attest to. Remember, I'm only one agent, and I can merely tell you about the lives of a few of my buddies, but there are armies of us out there. So don't think this is the whole story by any means.

Let's see, where should I begin, with the survivors or the casualties? This last case was the one that really turned my head around. I'll tell you about her. I've always been a sucker for high-spirited, cute 16 year old blondes. And this girl, Marin, had all it takes to make any creature's heart skip a beat. But Marin bit the dust, as the young kids say these days, a few weeks ago. What a heartbreaker. Her insatiable curiosity and zest for life was so impressive, her spirit so remarkable. She was special all right, and things will never be the same, not since Marin. Her death taught me every thing I ever feared about the consequences of over-reacting.

The day she died, a Saturday afternoon, lightning bolts kept flashing across the sky, but it wouldn't rain. Marin lived in a small Kansas town, known for its vicious tornadoes. She told her mother that she was headed for the bowling alley with a couple of her friends. Mrs. McDonald urged her to be careful because of the oncoming storm. Of course, Marin didn't like being treated like a little kid, so she wised off and gave her mom some static before she left.

"Mom, didn't I just have a birthday, you know, a year older, a year wiser? And haven't I always been real careful about any tornado warnings? When will you ever let me grow up? I love you Mom, but sometimes, you drive me nuts. You know J.J.'s has a shelter in case we need it, now I gotta go. Carrie's waiting for me."

"Okay, okay. Marin, go. I'll see you when you get home." By this time, Marin realized that she'd been a little too harsh on dear old Mom, so she tried to make up for it with a good-bye kiss.

"Bye Mom, I'll see you about five, okay?" She kissed her on the cheek and ran out the door.

Marin had been ill throughout her childhood and adolescence. She suffered from frequent episodes of hay fever, sinus problems, and stomach aches. With age, the predicament worsened. Minor headaches became major ones. Her mild gastrointestinal upsets grew more serious, and included bouts of acute abdominal pain.

A family physician, troubled by the increased severity decided it was time to consult a specialist. Marin was finally referred to an allergist. The appointment was only a few days away. Now if the hometown doctor had known about me, my enemies and my pals, that we were actually at the root of her problems, much of Marin's suffering could have been alleviated, and her life saved.

Our power, as antibodies, to either protect or destroy is frequently underestimated. Often, people tend to blame emotional problems. Like Marin, sometimes her mom and the doctor believed the complaints were a teenager's way of rebelling and gaining attention, or a method of playing hooky from school. Of course, the mind and body are both important to consider, but for people, even experts in the field of psychology, to deny my existence with so much obvious proof. Wise up.

Especially these days, we're busier than ever fighting off environmental stressors that hypersensitive people can't seem to adapt to.

I understand what some psychologists believe. The mind can be so influential in causing or combating disease. But so often, it's the misunderstanding and lack of proper education and health care that causes an unnecessary death of an allergic or asthmatic victim. Just like Marin, all she needed was a lifesaver kit, one shot of epinephrine and she might have made it to the hospital. Now all we can do is hopefully learn from our mistakes.

Anyway, Marin had allergies, severe ones. It was one of those cases where nobody paid any attention to them, me or my pals. I tried to pull out at the last minute when I realized it was too late, but the damage was done. It happened right on the floor of the bowling alley. A yellow jacket was the culprit. Don't ask me how it got inside, but there it flew, buzzing around as if it owned the place. Everyone began to squirm around, giggling and screaming like typical teenage girls, except for Marin. She wanted to take care of the problem so that the bowling could continue.

"You guys, it's just a dumb old bee. I'm gonna get a shoe and kill it. Carrie, give me your tennis shoe." Carrie reached under the seating area and looked for her shoe, but couldn't find it, so she tossed a sandal to Marin.

"Here. Be careful."

"There he is over on that chair! God, he's big. Oh, be careful, Marin, if you miss I hear they really get mad and come after you." One of the girls pointed and backed up.

"Okay. Here goes." She tiptoed over toward the yellow jacket and slammed the shoe down to squash it.

"Oh shoot, watch out I missed him. Stupid bee, moved right at the last minute. There he is. Watch out Debbie!" By this time the girls and several others were yelling and shuffling around, so the man at the front desk ran over and asked what the commotion was.

"I'm trying to kill this darn bee. Do you have a fly swatter? Maybe we could kill it that way ," Marin said.

"Marin, watch out, there he is on your back. Get him off, somebody!" Carrie yelled as she ran toward her.

"Ow! He stung me, get him off!" Marin screamed while swinging her arms.

"There, I got him," Carrie said as she stomped on the bee after it had fallen to the floor. "Come over here. Are you all right?" Her friends followed Marin as she went to sit down.

"Yeah, I guess I'm okay. That hurt though. Did you get the stupid bee? We should have just left him alone." She raised her shirt and asked Carrie to take a look at it. "Is it red, Carrie, or what?"

"Yes, it's red all right and it looks like it's swelling too. We better get you home."

But Marin never made it home. She never even made it to the door. The villain had struck an innocent victim. At that point it was our duty to step in and try to battle the poison. We were ready. My friends and I were always ready. That was the problem, we liked to fight, and we got so we did it too often and too viciously. Our intentions were good, but it didn't matter. Her immune system got out of hand and the poor kid died. Anaphylactic shock. She started breathing funny and I could actually see her muscle fibers tightening up. I told everyone to pull back, that we were fighting the antigen too much. But everything had gone haywire and I knew it was too late. She became unconscious and the next thing to go was her heart. What a scene, a sad story. She died, like I said, right there on the bowling alley floor.

You can see how terrible I feel. Here I am a do-gooder gone sour. Not that I haven't done my share of saving lives and helping people fight their allergies.

4

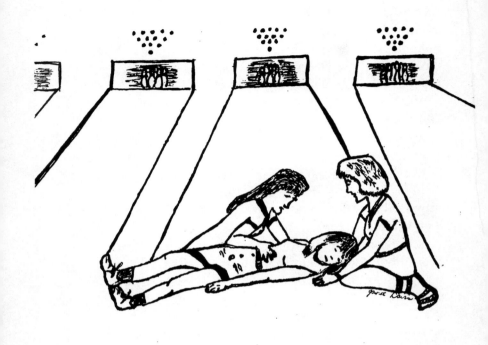

IN MEMORY OF MARIN
AND ALL
ALLERGIC VICTIMS
Illustration by Janet Davis

5

Believe me, the life of an antibody isn't the easiest, most flamboyant job in the world. But we lost her, and it certainly took its toll on me that day. So I decided to spill my guts, tell you the inside story, the nitty gritty about those creeps, the allergies.

Now if you're at all familiar with the life cycle of an antibody, you probably won't believe a word of any of this. Don't ask me why I'm still around, assigned to case after case. I lost many of my buddies when Marin died. I thought that's the way it worked, when the host dies, so do I. Maybe I'm destined to live out one scenario after another, until I get it right or until I've learned all I'm supposed to, I don't know. Maybe it's reincarnation. But if it is, I remember all of my past cases.

So if I tell you my story, what's in it for me? Well everything. Sometimes in a lifetime, animals, human beings, even fourth world creatures, as we're sometimes called; we all feel as if there is something we must do. Well, it's my turn. I've got to do it for Marin, for me, because if I don't, allergies will go on destroying people, and it's not fair, because they're really the bad guys, not us, the antibodies.

CHAPTER 2

Death isn't always the end result from an allergy attack. Marin's was certainly one of the most unfortunate cases I can recall. But believe me, allergies are permeating people's lives and causing a great deal of subtle, as well as obvious and profound physical and mental distress. They have got to be stopped.

I remember one young couple who lived in Akron, Ohio. Tim and Barb knew the essence of love, at least for the first few years anyway. Oh, everyone knew that sooner or later they'd be forced to come down to Earth with their ideal love. But, I know the inside story and one of the main causes of their marital deterioration. Barb endured significant allergies which constantly toyed with her body and caused all sorts of reactions. We fought them for years, but could not get rid of them. She experienced an assortment of adverse effects, from ugly cold sores, nausea and ulcer-like symptoms, to painful migraines and an increasingly despondent nature. She began to lose her pizzazz and consequently, Tim began to lose interest. One night they had a big fight.

"Go to the New Year's party without me. I don't care, I don't feel good anyway," Barb said sarcastically.

"That's the problem, you never feel good. I'm sorry, but I'm tired of hearing about it. And we can't afford anymore of those tests. We're running out of money just because you never feel well. And I can't sit around and baby-sit you, because I want to live a happy life. Do you know what that means, a happy life? Remember when we were happy?" Tim hurried toward the front door.

Of course Barb burst into tears. "Go out and have fun. You deserve it." She wiped the tears from her eyes. "But so do I, and it's not fair. It's not my fault that I'm sick again. I'm trying as hard as I can." She walked over to the sink in the kitchen to get a glass of water and a tissue or

7

paper towel to blow her nose. "That's all, just go. Oh, I hate it, I hate it. I hate being sick!" She cried uncontrollably and hit her fist on the table as she sat back down.

"You're just getting to be a nagging neurotic, that's all there is to it. I'm sorry sweetheart, but I'm not letting your problems spoil my New Years. Now if you want to get dressed, we'll go together, otherwise I'm leaving right now." He looked directly at her and awaited an answer.

"Go. Just go. I can't. I feel terrible." So he left and slammed the door behind him. Afterward, Barb took two Aspirins, two tablespoons of Pepto Bismol, turned the radio on, climbed into bed feeling alienated, guilty and hurt, and cried herself to sleep.

The friction kept worsening between the two "lovebirds" because of Barb's poor health, and their marriage began to crumble. However, fortunately in this case, Barb's doctor soon recommended a specialist, an internist, who in turn referred her to an allergist. After a comprehensive physical and mental examination, some scrutinizing of her medical history and allergy tests, the doctor concluded that Barb definitely had some allergy related medical problems. They were so thrilled to finally have some answers.

Within three months time, she was aware of many of the causes of her illness. The couple moved from the damp, moldy basement apartment which they had been living in, and obtained the help of a qualified nutritionist. Barb stopped taking Aspirin and an oral contraceptive which she found had caused some of her reactions. In time she began an exercise program and gradually began to feel healthier. After awhile, she lost the nervousness and fatigue which had accompanied her debilitated condition. Barb and Tim soon found their marriage to be happily intact once again.

That's one inspiring story about a marriage that survived an allergy affliction. Unfortunately, thousands of others have failed under similar circumstances, not solely because someone in the family had an allergy, but in many cases, partly because of it. Allergies create stress, and stress creates allergies. Those allergy creeps like to take advantage of bodies with lowered resistance. On the other hand, so many times they're responsible for lowering the resistance, especially when an individual can't manage to obtain adequate rest. So there you have it, the vicious cycle.

CHAPTER 3

Swelling is one of the reactions that allergies like to cause. And it's something they do very well. Once they attack, we try to fight back, then a chemical called histamine is released and swelling occurs.

One of the worst places for this phenomenon to take place is within the hearing apparatus. It happened one time to Kevin, a little boy I liked. There is another sad truth to this story. I was partially to blame for causing Kevin's deafness.

Only five at the time, he was a very amiable little guy. His mom came home from the allergist's office one day, with the, luckily, not so bad news. She would not have known how to break it to her husband or Kevin if the answer was no again, the deafness irreparable. The allergist had finally found a surgeon who could help. Eventually Kevin would be able to hear again.

Mrs. Koleski sat down at the dinner table one night and explained what the doctor told her. "Dr. Bates says that Kevin's hearing loss is correctable. Thank God. We'll continue to treat this latest infection, but as soon as it clears up we can try the surgery. He assured me that it's going to be okay. You're going to be all right Kevin." She stood up and walked over to her son, hugged him, and then made the appropriate gestures to help him understand what she was saying. Kevin said the first thing he wanted to hear again was his cartoons. The three of them cried and hugged each other.   Later that evening, Mr. and Mrs. Koleski sat up in bed talking to each other, expressing both guilt and relief.

"Why? How did we let him get this bad? Why didn't we get to the cause of it sooner? Why?" questioned Mrs. Koleski.

"I don't know dear, that's a very good question." He looked up toward the ceiling, then leaned his head over

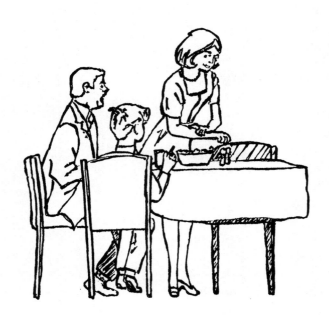

on his wife's shoulder. "I don't know why. We just kept thinking he would get better. Kev doesn't deserve this. We've learned our lesson. From now on, we take his allergies very seriously. We'll watch him really close. Okay honey? He's going to be all right." They embraced. Within minutes they were both asleep. Tomorrow they could begin to move away from their nightmare.

Shortly before six, the alarm clock beeped loudly. After realizing their good fortune, the beauty of something called a "second chance," the Koleskis both stared at each other and smiled. The sun glistened through the silk curtains and a cool, soft breeze swept across their faces. But the sound emitting from the television in the living room reminded them, too quickly, that their deaf son sat watching the early morning cartoons unable to hear the animated voices of Bugs Bunny and the Smurfs. He'll hear them again soon. Thank God, just a little longer, Kev, they both thought to themselves.

Do you see how it works? Allergies are the antagonists. We just try to counter-attack. Trouble is, there is a fine line between protecting and maintaining an equilibrium within the human body and the other extreme of causing an all out war, a hyper-reaction.

CHAPTER 4

It's remarkable what the human body can tolerate. I've been involved with the heavy drinkers, modern-day pot heads, cocaine sniffers, food addicts, smokers, and the caffeine and sugar extremists. And every time I enter into a specific case, I say to myself, Don't you know there's a war going on inside here? Have some mercy! Give us a break! Things begin to break down and no antibody in the world should be subjected to the kind of torture or workload people throw at us. The sad part is that they don't know how lucky they are. If they'd just wise up and think about how important there health is. But then, who am I to judge humans? I know they have their "grounds of existence," just like we do. Like all of the black lung or asbestosis cases. Maybe sometimes, socio-economic reasons make it necessary that some people work certain jobs which cause these deadly diseases. But when it's a matter of life and breath, all I keep thinking about is that there's got to be another way. There's just got to.

It's sad enough when the innocent victims get sick, but the self-destructive ones who have a choice and take part in digging their own premature graves, those cases simply flabbergast me. You'd think that by now, Americans, the French, Germans, Italians, Russians, Indians, Mexicans, all different cultures and species would possess some sophisticated, sound, basic knowledge about their bodies and minds in regards to feeling healthy.

Then there's the other side of the coin, too, the one that drives me half crazy. That's the "supplemented" generation. I'm referring to the individual who can't stop thinking about health. With adequate health education, seems like it should happen naturally, easily, if people follow basic principles. Not so much an obsession. I suppose everyone has to find their own way and I don't discredit anyone's willingness and desire to search.

Sometimes, though, I just feel like there is too much talk and not enough action. After Eastern philosophies, nutrition fads and a multitude of various supplements and ideologies to escape the responsibility of coming right back to where people started, namely themselves; where does the individual go then? That's my question.

It's the ones making a sincere effort to get well or remain healthy that I care about. People like Marin, Barb, the Koleskis and Captain Ramon Rodz, a navy pilot who needed my help for awhile.

We flew over deserts, oceans, wastelands, mountains, vast prairies, countries and all over the United States. He knew how to handle a plane the way a Pope guides a congregation through a prayer, smoothly, serenely, and with never-ending courage and reassurance. Captain Rodz was the best. I'm not going to elaborate here on another case of mine gone haywire, so don't worry. On the contrary, the Captain had everything under control and his life was something to marvel at. I think he even slept with a good sense of humor and purpose in mind.

But he wasn't immune to occasional problems, and one particular thing was beginning to annoy him. For about the last month, every time he flew, approximately an hour or so after take off, he started sneezing. He experienced tightness in his chest, itched, felt lethargic and nauseous and also suffered from mild visual blurring and an annoying ringing in his ears.

Since Captain Rodz was well aware of all the lives he was responsible for, as he readied for take off one day, he vowed to himself that he would not fly again until the cause for his disconcerting symptoms was discovered. Fortunately, the physician suspected an allergy, so it didn't take long to find the culprit.

"First, Captain, let me assure you that your physical exam results were fine, nothing out of the ordinary or any specific reasons for your symptoms showed up. But that's common in cases like this. I realize however, that you do have some type of unique problem that could be very dangerous in your line of work. Now I'm going to ask you to try to be specific as I ask you some questions," the doctor explained.

"Go right ahead Doctor, that's why I'm here. I'll do my best." He crossed his legs and leaned back in the chair.

"Okay. I want you to tell me if you can think of any strong odors which you are aware of each time you enter the plane or cockpit. Can you think of any scents which stand out?" he asked.

"Well, let's see, I never really thought about it. I think a few of the flight attendants wear perfume, but nothing very distinguishable. And I do smell a certain type of cleansing agent, occasionally, on the instrument board. But, it doesn't seem to bother me. Other than that, I can't really think of anything."

"That's good, exactly the type of things I need to know. Now, tell me what you usually eat the night before a flight. I'm especially looking for a favorite food or one that you eat regularly before each flight." The captain began to laugh, but then regained his serious, cooperative self.

"Oh Lord, what do I eat? It varies so much. My wife, Sherry, makes a delicious lasagna dinner on certain nights when I'm home," Captain Rodz answered.

Dr. Wilson uncrossed his arms and smiled. He sat in a brown leather chair and leaned forward with a pen in his hand ready to write down everything mentioned.

"I'll tell you Doctor, my main dinners in the evening usually consist of chicken, fish occasionally, usually perch, a good T-bone steak and some Italian or Mexican food. In Phoenix, Arizona I have a favorite Chinese restaurant, usually it's chicken and broccoli. My other favorite vegetables are corn, fried okra and cauliflower with cheese sauce and salads. I do eat a lot of salads with vinegar and

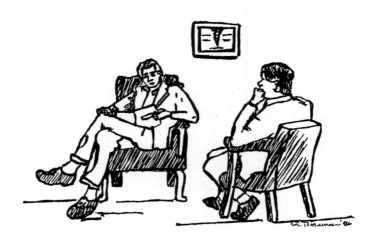

oil.   I don't eat shrimp because of a severe reaction once."

"Very good. Now, can you think of anything else?" asked Dr. Wilson.

"I think that's about it."

The phone rang and interrupted their detective work for a few minutes. Then the doctor persisted and wanted to know about desserts, beverages and breakfast selections.

"Oh, for desserts, let's see, that would be cheesecake, Sherry's homemade apple cobbler, or orange sherbet when I'm on the road. For breakfast, that's simple, scrambled eggs, bacon, toast, a glass of orange juice and plenty of black coffee."

"How much coffee do you drink?"

"Usually about three cups, but I switched to decaffeinated awhile back because I was getting some headaches." After a short pause, Captain Rodz continued to disclose more dietary information. "And I do drink a couple beers occasionally or some ice tea or water."

"Do you drink much milk or pop?" asked Dr. Wilson. "No, I never cared that much for either." He shook his head no.

"Okay, now, can you think of anything else, particularly anything unusual you've been eating lately, something you don't ordinarily..."

The Captain interrupted. "Wait a minute, there is something I've been eating lately that I don't usually eat, for the last month or so. Doctor, I think you're a genius. Is it possible to have the kind of symptoms I've been having from eating a lot of walnuts?"

"It's possible, Captain. Some people do have specific serious allergies to peanuts or walnuts." Both men smiled and realized that they had probably just finished their little game of Sherlock Holmes and Dr. Watson. "Are you eating them prior to flying or the night before or what?" asked the Doctor.

"Let me tell you how I got hooked on them. Peggy, a new neighbor from next door, apparently buys a bulk quantity of nuts wholesale each month and then ends up selling them. My wife has been buying walnuts and peanuts and stuffing them in my pockets and suitcase before I leave home. And, I keep eating more and more each flight. I've gotten used to them, is that it Doctor?" the Captain asked inquisitively.

"Well, we won't know for sure until we administer some tests, but it certainly sounds possible. I'd like you to go down to the second floor, to the allergy testing lab and ask for Dr. Teller, and we'll find out. He's waiting for you. I told him you'd be down sometime this afternoon. They'll also pull your chart and take a good look at it. In the meantime, don't eat any more nuts. I think we might be getting there." He stood up and offered to shake the Captain's hand.

They shook hands and exchanged smiles as Captain Rodz thanked the doctor, then turned to walk out the door.

"Now they'll fill you in on all of the details downstairs. If I can be of any more help, let me know," said Dr. Wilson.

They had figured it out. As soon as the Captain refrained from eating the daily walnuts, the physical symptoms which had become such a nuisance and potential occupational and health hazard, subsided and finally disappeared.

A word of caution, here, if I might, what the Doctor said is true, some people have food allergies. But this is another controversial matter which drives me half crazy. On one hand, there are people out there with legitimate food intolerances, allergic victims who suffer for years because the cause of their disruptive bodily reactions cannot be detected. Then there are actually children and/or adults starving or panicking at the sight of anything edible, because they have been frightened into believing that they are allergic to everything. In other words, to survive, the individual would actually be forced to live in a protective shield of some sort.

Dr. Coballan, a specialist in food allergies, cautions people to determine legitimate food reactions in an objective way, not to overreact, and remember how important nutrition can be to health. He wrote a book on the subject.

CHAPTER 5

As I said before, I've been around, and one of the places where I've spent a lot of time is in the school classroom. From the west coast to the east, up to Canada, throughout the midwestern and southern states, into Europe, and all around the globe, antibodies are prevalent residents. Allergy is a common cause of infancy and childhood disorders. What bothers me about the area of disease is the fact that despite all of our endeavors to make it clear that allergies are the antagonists, so often, nobody pays attention.

Consequently, allergies and asthma frequently become two of the most unattended and devastating developmentally disabling diseases known to the human race. The magnitude of the damage to the human spirit and potential resulting from allergic and asthmatic diseases, may never be fully realized. Not only physical damage, but some emotional or sociological damage can result as well, partially because any disease affects all facets of a person's life. Allergies and asthma, and all of the debilitating side effects which accompany these diseases, are quite often not obvious to human eyesight or perceptibility, the way other handicaps might be.

But, trust me, the asthmatic or allergic sufferer is grateful for the reversible nature of symptoms and the healthy days experienced, the days or hours when, although vulnerable, they can still enjoy life in a healthy way.

Statistics? If you really want to hear the facts, I've got lots of figures. I'm talking millions of afflicted people, and millions of lost days from school, work and life in general.

I could go on and on, all of the interesting people I've known, humans from all walks of life, including celebrities, brilliant inventors, artists, and musicians, the athletes. I even tried to help a President once, but his medical friends never seemed to make the connection and failed to get to the source of the problem, even after all the alarms we set off. He suffered so needlessly. I'd like to talk about that case, but I'm afraid I'm due on another one, a follow-up, someone I've known for a long time, but left on her own a few years back, because she didn't need me anymore.

I want to see how Sara's doing, see if she finally resolved everything. She wrote about her life too, a book called *Gone with the Tires*, in which she tells about her bicycle touring trip along the Pacific Coast. It meant a lot to her because she was an asthmatic who had struggled with allergies all her life. I suppose it was Sara's turning point.

Can this actually be the girl I used to know? She looks healthier than ever. Her journeys through life and health education studies must have paid off. But, I always knew she was a fighter, that's why I left earlier than usual. She was making all the right moves, so I figured she'd obtain quality health sooner or later.

It looks like she's on vacation, at home with her relatives in Indiana. Everything looks good, this could be fun. It'll be nice to be back in the swing of live action again, and not pulling everything from memory. Besides, I could use a vacation and some fun myself, as long as I'm getting my point across.

CHAPTER 6

Toss me a cigarette, Stacy, and your lighter," Sara requested. The two young women sat across from each other at a dining room table.

"No. My sister does not smoke," Stacy professed as she grabbed the package of Marlboro Lights and held onto them tightly.

"C'mon. I'm tired of being different. I won't inhale, it's just my way of adapting, relaxing and not letting the smoke get to my head or my lungs." The two of them wrestled until Sara managed to free the package of cigarettes from Stacy's hands. "I know as long as I'm visiting, I'd better get used to the smoke."

"No!" Stacy persisted.

"Yes! I just want to have one, okay." Sara put the cigarette in her mouth and lit it, began to puff on it and emit smoke into the air. "See, no big deal." Stacy started to laugh and shook her head in disbelief.

"You've changed."

"Why, what do you mean?" Sara smiled.

"I don't think you should be smoking. That's not you at all. It used to be all you'd do is come back here and complain about it to Mom or Dad or me." Stacy looked surprised again as Sara took another puff.

"I know, huh. Well, I'll tell you something Stacy. It took me a lot of years to learn how to be healthy because of that dumb asthma and my allergies. But once I did gain my health, I kept on going and going until I felt as if I had reached a point where nothing could hurt me, if I didn't let it. I mean, I still believe in certain basics regarding health. And, I found out the hard way a couple of times when I ran out of my inhaler, just how dangerous it is to be careless when two puffs can save my life. But for the most part, I feel so healthy now, not much can get my resistance down anymore." Finally, Sara took two quick puffs and put the cigarette out.

Stacy stood up and walked away from the kitchen table to see what her young son Tommy wanted.

"Mom, can I play over at Holly's on the swing set?"

"Is Holly home?" Stacy asked as she bent down to tie Tommy's tennis shoe.

"Yeah. She's right here, right there," he pointed, "in the front yard."

"Okay, but where's your sister? Is she still next door?"

"Yeah, she is. Bye." He ran out the door. Stacy walked to the refrigerator and opened the door to the freezing compartment. She dropped ice cubes into the green Tupperware glasses and filled them to the top with pink lemonade.

"Bye Tommy," Sara yelled from the front doorway. "Stacy, I'll turn the music back on. Let's listen to that one song again. What time's Hank coming home?"

"I think about five. He went to see about his job that starts tomorrow. So are you going up to Mom and Dad's later?" She handed a glass to Sara as they both sat down.

"Thanks. Yeah, I think I will. I was having fun the other night playing bartender and pool. I was winning at pool. I have to go get my quarters from my shorts, for the jukebox. Do you guys want to come tonight? Any possibility that Hank's mom and dad would baby-sit?"

"No! They sure won't if they know we're going to the bar. They take 'em on Saturday nights, though, so maybe we can go then."

"Okay, sounds good. Oh no, look at the time, I better get ready to go. I want to catch Dad before he leaves." She walked toward the bedroom, almost tripped over the toy collie that scratched vigorously in the hallway.

Sara stopped momentarily to comb her hair in the bathroom.

"Hey Stacy, have you seen my yellow shorts? They aren't where I left them!" She shouted from the bedroom doorway.

"Oh, um," she paused, "try under the bed, the kids were playing in there this morning."

"All right." Sara lifted the disheveled covers from the bed and shook them to see if the shorts were intermingled between the sheet and the bedspread, then looked under the bed to no avail. She grabbed the bedpost and slid the bed to the left slightly and heard the quarters jingling. "There you are," she said and unsnapped the two pockets on the right and transferred a handful of quarters from her shorts to her jacket pocket.

"Stacy, listen," Sara walked toward the kitchen, "if Dave should call, tell him I'll be at Mom's in the morning so he can call over there, okay. We're supposed to go sailing tomorrow."

"Oh, you're gonna stay at Mom and Dad's tonight?"

"Yeah, I think so, rather than driving all the way back over here."

"Okay, I'll tell him." She moved toward Sara to give her a hug.

"Ah-choo! Oh my stupid nose." Sara reached for the paper towels on a counter top to the left.

"What's the matter?"

"Oh you know, it's my sneezing season again. My nose and eyes have been acting up since last week. Had to take an antihistamine this morning and I was okay for awhile, but now it's acting up again. I hate to take them because they make me sleepy," Sara sniffled.

"I heard on the news today that it's the height of the hay fever season. Hank's been having trouble too."

"Sure is. Guess I'll have to survive it as usual though, that's all. How's his asthma been lately?"

While Sara inched her way toward the front door after making sure she had her purse, Stacy explained that Hank was much better since he left his job at the chemical plant. She inhaled on a cigarette, then turned to avoid blowing the smoke toward Sara.

"Well listen Stacy, I better get going. It is so good to see you and talking with you again. God I miss everyone so much. You know we have the neatest, most loving family there is. I may just have to move back here in a couple of years. The thing is, Colorado feels like home too. I'm always split between two homes, here and there. I sure am healthier there though, with the dry climate, you know."

"I know Sara, but we miss you a lot and it is nice to have you around." Stacy smiled.

"Well, we'll see. Then I'll see you tomorrow evening, sometime, right?" She gave Stacy a hug.

"Sure. That'll be great. See ya later, and have fun." As Sara walked out the front door, she smiled back at her sister, then several children began to say hello and ask if they could go for a ride in her truck. "Well, sorry, "I have to go somewhere right now, but maybe tomorrow, okay?"

Later at the bar, Sara sat on a barstool and listened to some loud country-western tunes that played on the jukebox, while she talked to her dad.

"I saw Laura and Bill today, and their five kids. She lives in a beautiful house out in Chesterton, and she has a forest for a front and back yard. Really Dad, it's a nice old country-type house and her kids are so neat." Sara glanced toward the pool table and then quickly turned her head back toward her father.

"Oh. That's great. Laura. Do I know her? Oh, now I remember, the one with the long hair, your friend from high school," he said as he turned to ask the couple at the end of the bar if they would like another beer. "Just a second." He walked around the corner where the beer was stocked and got out two Old Styles, opened them quickly,

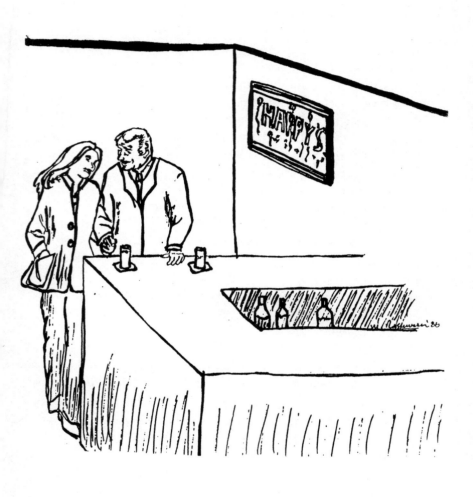

set them down in front of the two customers, and then rang up two dollars on the cash register.

He walked back to Sara. "So they live in Chesterton? What road is that off of, if the house is located in the country?"

"You just exit the toll road off of Route 19, about three fourths of a mile turn left on the road before the viaduct and they're right down the street on the left, but they're hidden behind a bunch of trees," explained Sara.

"Hmm. It sounds nice. I think I know that area. So you've been visiting everyone and having a good time, huh? Have you seen Dave? When are you two gonna get back together?" Her father asked. "I know you still love each other."

"We're supposed to go sailing tomorrow," replied Sara. "Dad, we're friends, and I'll always love him, that's all I can say. Everything has just changed so much, what we had is in the past." She turned and looked to see who walked in the door.

"Hi Mitch, how are ya?" Sara's dad headed back to the end of the bar again to get Mitch his usual to drink.

A red-haired lady sat at the other end of the bar and remarked, "There he is, Mitch the Magic Man." She turned toward the man who sat next to her, "This guy is good, honey, watch what he can do. Mitch, do the cigarette trick."

"I'm not doin' any tricks until I get me a cold beer, then I shall perform. John, where's my beer at?" The young man with wavy brown hair asked.

"Sure Mitch, here it is." John set the Miller's down, then rang it up.

"Hey, I know that guy," said a gray-haired, middle-aged man in a blue overall suit, standing at the bar. "He's the one who got his belly button cut off in Vietnam." A burst of laughter sounded throughout the bar, following the remark.

"You have a rowdy crowd in here sometimes, don't you?" Sara whispered to her father as she leaned toward him.

"Yes. we do, we really do." he nodded. "Listen Sara, you're mother should be here any second, and Julie to take my place. We're going out to dinner, you're coming along, aren't you?"

"Sure. That's why I'm here, to spend time with you guys."

"Well that's what we'll do as soon as she gets here."

"Great Dad." Sara reached into her pocket for a few more quarters because the music had stopped, and she wanted to liven the place up again.

Now see, this is what I don't like about this job. Just when I start having fun or getting to like the people I'm around, I'm expected to drop everything and I'm required to jump right into a more challenging and less leisurely situation. At least I know that things worked out pretty good for Sara. When I think about how she almost died so many times, or how easily she could have ended up on an oxygen tank, or sneezing and wheezing her life away, because of her asthma and allergies. But she's not, she's got the control now. It makes me feel proud. Oh well, when duty calls. Another emergency I guess.

CHAPTER 7

Where am I anyway? What is this place? Let me look at my orders. I'm stationed back in Denver now. Several people are lounging in beige, cushioned chairs, scanning magazines. I'm watching two young children play with bright-colored toys in the corner, and one woman is just staring into space. A small framed man, confined to a wheelchair with tubing in his nose and an oxygen tank at his side just told a joke to his wife and a nurse.

The nurse tried to look interested, but obviously, she has other things on her mind. She laughed at the punch line and then excused herself, picked up a chart from a basket on the receptionist's desk and walked into a square-shaped room. Another nurse listened carefully as she took a patient's blood pressure.

"Mrs. Beller, we just need to get one more thing now. You know how to do this, right?" The nurse reached to assist the patient.

"Oh yes," she said as she stood up slowly, holding onto the nurse's shoulder. "I've done it plenty of times. Just let me catch my breath first. I had a rough night last night with my attack."

"Okay, you just take your time, whenever you're ready. Stand right up here, just a little closer, and I'll put a chair behind you."

"Right here?" Mrs. Beller asked. As she tried to catch her breath, wheezing sounds became audible.

"You are having a rough time today, aren't you? Yes, that's fine. Now, let me put this in here and hand this to you whenever you're ready. Remember, blow as hard and as long as you can," explained the nurse.

"All right," agreed Mrs. Beller. She placed the circular-shaped cardboard mouthpiece into her mouth, took a deep breath, held her hand on her chest and exhaled into the device.

"And blow, blow, blow, keep going, keep going. Good, a little longer. Good, that's it!" the nurse said enthusiastically. The patient's face reddened while she coughed harshly. The nurse cautiously watched Mrs. Beller and offered her a Kleenex.

"Here. Are you all right now? Just relax a minute. You know it makes people cough like that."

"Oh I'm fine now. It's just for a little bit, I just can't help it, it makes me cough." Mrs. Beller blew her nose again.

"Now, let me see if Dr. Loy is ready to see you. I'll be right back." The nurse walked down a hallway, wrote something next to Mrs. Beller's name on a piece of paper, wrote the patient's name and the doctor's name on an erasable schedule board, and then returned to the work-up room where the patient sat waiting.

"Okay, Mrs. Beller follow me, right down here to room four and Dr. Loy will be right in." They walked toward the room. The nurse put Mrs. Beller's chart in a holder outside the door on the wall.

"Just have a seat, and he'll be right in," she smiled.

"All right, thank you." Mrs. Beller laid her purse down next to the chair.

Well, I figured out where I am. It's obvious that I'm in an allergy/respiratory clinic of some sort. Look at these charts, sinus infections, asthma, food sensitivity, allergies, immune diseases, and those people out there, now it's really getting crowded with patients looking for some relief. The anguish on their faces, the tissues in their hands, and the familiar mature attitude of acceptance, even from the kids. I've seen it all so many times before. At least these days there are clinics like this one to rehabilitate them, give them hope and a way to work toward a healthier existence.

This assignment is unusual for me. I'm usually on a one to one basis, but there are allergic and asthmatic sufferers all over this place that could use my assistance. Evidently I'm here as an observer, because I'm inside this one nurse, not a patient. That's fine with me. The work that needs to be done here looks overwhelming anyway.

But I'm sure I'm here for some important reason. Something is in store for me, I'd make a fifty dollar bet on that. I think I'll head up toward the blood lines and see if any of my old buddies are anywhere in the near vicinity.

CHAPTER 8

"Our duty, our mission will remain the same: to serve, protect and preserve mankind through advanced biomedical endeavors in the areas of immunological medicine. You have played an essential role in providing information on immune-deficiency, allergic and autoimmune diseases. Above all, tonight, you are saluted for your devotion toward humanitarian goals." As the speech ended, the high-ranking antibody stepped down from the diaphragmatic stage, the crowd dispersed, and everyone headed back to their plasmic living quarters.

"George, is that you?" I asked.

"Henry, my God, you son of a gun, what the heck are you doing here?" George asked. We exchanged affectionate grins.

"Just got here, you know how the boss works, right smack dab in the middle of some fun, back in the midwest, and the next thing I know, my papers are in and here I am. What's the situation look like anyway? Well, never mind for now, you can tell me later. Tell me how life's been treating you."

"Oh, things are pretty good. Can't complain. My luck's been all right, not too many sad cases, some minor arthritic ones, most of them have been real promising. Just got off of one of those adolescent cases, you know how they can go downhill fast, if someone doesn't work with 'em. J.D. had the works: allergies, asthma, emotional problems, learning difficulties, a doomed to fail attitude. You name it, he had it all. But that young man shaped up so fast once he enrolled in a school for learning disabled kids. He started trusting his teachers and realized they weren't trying to take his individuality away, only give him a chance, so he could start getting some education. Of course, the saddest case I had was a thirty-six year old woman with the big one, AIDS. She hung in there for years, but then she died. So anyway, how about you? What's this about the midwest?" George looked at me with his usual curious manner.

"Oh, had to go see about a follow-up. Remember Sara, the one with all the allergies and asthma when she was growing up, back in the fifties and sixties? The one allergic to aspirin, watermelon but she ate it anyway and her mom and dad smoked?"

"Sure I remember Sara, loved to run but always had trouble in gym class and used to take us to the movies all the time, had the hay fever in the summer, cold sores and asthma attacks. You sure did spend a lot of time with that girl. How's it looking for her nowadays, okay?" George asked.

"Well, all right for the most part, but do you know what that character was doing? Smoking!"

"Smoking? That's impossible, the way she used to yell at her mom and dad and brother. Are you kidding me?"

(I knew George would not believe it.) "I'm not fooling you. She only smoked one time at her sister's house, but she was definitely smoking. Said she wouldn't inhale, but she was tired of being different, and it was her way of letting go of the fear of cigarette smoke. Explained she felt so well, nothing could bother her anymore."

"Well," remarked George, "maybe she was just trying to prove a point or something." He paused.

"Could be, thing is, I know her. She's got a dog, you know, and sometimes she thinks she can just deny her potentially allergic condition, and then she gets run down and the asthma flairs," I explained.

"Know what you mean, it happens all the time, but you know what, I'd rather see her react that way. This is my own personal opinion now, but I'd rather see her do that than act like she's afraid of everything. Remember that one family, the Roberts and how they sold their little boy's bike because he had asthma. His grandfather tried to tell them to keep it, but they sold it and the boy kept failing after that, anything new he'd try, he just kept deteriorating, and got weaker everyday. Had to spend so much time alone because the other kids didn't want to play with him. You see my point?" asked George.

I nodded and concluded in agreement that Sara possibly knew exactly what she was doing. But I thought to myself how sick and frail some asthmatics are when they really get debilitated. A smoke-filled room or puffing off of a cigarette could be ludicrous for someone like that. I also said to myself, I hope Sara quits playing around and just stays away from smoke as much as possible.

"Listen, Henry, it's good to see ya, lets go and we'll sit down and have a bite to eat and talk for awhile. I hate to do it, but we better talk some business, too. Have you been informed about anything yet, what's going on inside this nurse's body?"

"No, I just got in today. I was supposed to talk to the guy who spoke tonight, but you can bring me up to date on the inside story. I'll go and see him tomorrow," I smiled.

"Sure. Yeah, I have to talk to you. I'm glad you're going to be here with us. We can use your strategic mind and your experience."

"Sounds like war again, am I right?" I asked, almost afraid of the affirmative.

"Well, that's the possibility," George sighed.

"You mean likelihood," I replied.

"Come on, follow me, let's go get food and then some rest. Hey, I'll bet I have some news that you're unaware of, that'll just knock you off your feet," George chuckled.

"What?" I raised my eyebrows.

"Females, that's what, they've infiltrated, say we have about two hundred in this district alone and thousands throughout."

But I told George I had him on this one. I had been working too, not sitting idle in some retirement camp, and I let him know I enjoyed women, their company and their intelligence. We grabbed some food and took it back to his headquarters. He wanted to talk about the serious stuff, what might occur and how we had to prepare, but I made him take a detour. So we just sat there and talked mostly about our success cases from the past.

CHAPTER 9

"The first thing we need to do Ellie, to treat your sinusitis, is to open the passages that drain the sinus areas," said Dr. Wicker.

"How do you do that? Does it hurt?" asked Ellie, a soft-spoken, shy ten year old brunette.

"No, it can usually be done with decongestant medications and by breathing steam from a vaporizer. Then if that doesn't make it completely better, we have other methods that we can try. And drinking lots of water, can you do that Ellie?" coaxed the doctor.

"Uh huh. But what are sinuses and how do they get plugged up Doctor?" Ellie asked in a nasal tone as she twirled the ends of her long, brown curly hair with her fingers.

The doctor explained that she had something called an eth-moid sinus problem. Think of a sinus as a little cave or opening and eth-moid is just a name for one specific area.

"It's about right here." Dr. Wicker pointed as she touched Ellie near the nose. "And if it gets congested or filled up with a bunch of stuff, you know, that stuff you have to keep blowing your nose to get rid of, well, then it can cause pain between the eyes and make your eyelids swell, like they are."

The doctor glanced toward Ellie's mother who sat next to her daughter. "And we think Mrs. Gibner, that in Ellie's case, as you suspected, the sinus condition may require getting her allergies under better control. So we have a lot of work to do. But Ellie, we know what to do to start making you feel better, okay." She touched her softly on the right shoulder. At that moment a nurse standing near the door explained that there was a phone call for the doctor.

Dr. Wicker stood up, "All right, we were just about through here." The doctor asked the nurse to explain where the pharmacy was located and how the out patient clinic worked in relation to allergy testing and management, and to schedule another appointment in a week for Ellie. "Then I'll see you two in a week. Mrs. Gibner, if she doesn't begin to improve in a few days, or if you have any questions, just call."

Mrs. Gibner quickly thanked Dr. Wicker. As he began to leave, he reminded her to push the liquids, "unsweetened preferably." Then he turned back and said, "Ellie, we're on the right track now, the medicine should help you feel better."

"Okay, bye."

While Clara, the nurse, explained a few things and answered some questions for Mrs. Gibner, a hospital aid in a blue, lengthy jacket walked by trying to find the clinic coordinator. "Excuse me," he said, "I'm from supplies and this is supposed to go to one of the pediatric nurses, is that you?" Clara accepted the box of respiratory supplies and said thank you.

When she finished up with Mrs. Gibner and Ellie, Clara walked down to the work-up room to see the next patient. Tammy managed the phones and the time schedule board, while Clara picked up a chart from the basket, looked at the name in the right hand corner and struggled to pronounce it. "Mister Dru-, Druserenski," Clara said as she looked at two men in business suits, and a woman and her two kids, who sat in chairs waiting to hear their names, along with several other asthmatics. One man stood up.

"Dru-ser-enski, how do you like that for a name?" He laughed.

"Oh it sounds all right. It's different." Clara smiled as the man walked toward her. "Would you follow me please?" gestured Clara.

"Certainly," he replied co-operatively.

"Just have a seat and take off your shoes please, so we can get your weight." He leaned down to untie his shoes. Clara glanced through the chart quickly to find the page that she needed and then asked, "Is this your first time here, Mr. Druserenski?"

"Yes it is. My doctor recommended this clinic and some of the education classes."

"Well good." She paused while she searched the room for her stethoscope. "Since this is your first time here, what we do in this room is weigh you, take your pulse and blood pressure and have you take a spirometry test. Now, I'll show you how to do that. It gives us an idea of what your breathing capacity is. Then, I'll see if the doctor is ready to see you."

"Oh, okay," he said.

"And you're here to see doctor who?" Clara asked.

"Dr. Loy," the patient answered. Clara checked to see what room number Dr. Loy occupied and wrote it in the lower left hand corner, along with the date, time, her initials and made a check mark by outpatient and spirometry test. "Now I need your age."

"Forty-eight," he replied matter-of-factly.

"And have you used an inhaler recently?"

"Yes, let's see, oh, about 11:00, no 11:30 this morning, I remember, just before I ate something." He patted his pudgy stomach.

Clara logged in the time, then said, "Step right up here."

Mr. Druserenski stepped up on the scale.

"It looks like 88.6 kilograms which is," she looked up at the conversion chart on the wall, "195 pounds."

The patient seemed puzzled at the reality of gaining a few pounds. The nurse told him to have a seat and put his shoes back on. Then she reached out and took a hold of his right hand. "Let me get your pulse." She placed her index and middle finger over his radial pulse and listened while looking at the second hand on her watch. After fifteen seconds passed, she jotted down seventy-six.

Next, Clara maneuvered a blood pressure cuff around Mr. Druserenski's right, upper arm. With her stethoscope in place, she pumped the black rubber bulb, then released it slowly until she heard a thump. She made a mental note of the systolic number. When she no longer heard the pulsating sound, she deflated the cuff, unravelled it, put the stethoscope back around her neck and then wrote down the two numbers.

"That's 124 over 76," Clara said. "Looks fine, not a high blood pressure at all."

"Well, that's about right for me." He sounded reassured.

"Is it?" Clara asked as she folded the cuff.

"Yes, I usually run about 126 or 130."

"Now I need you to do one more thing. Have you ever taken the spirometer test before?" Clara asked.

"Yes I know how to do it, but this one looks a little different than the one they used at St. Peter's Hospital. I just take a deep breath, right, and blow?" He inhaled and exhaled.

"That's right. You want to take a real deep breath, blow as hard and as long as you can. Here, you hold this, wait and let me put this on your nose and this in here. All right, we're all set."

Mr. Druserenski breathed deeply, pursed his lips over the circular shaped mouth piece and blew into it. Afterward he coughed and remarked in a weak voice, almost a whisper, "That hurts, you know."

"Does it? You mean your lungs as you breathed deeply?" Clara placed her hand on his chest.

"Yeah, there's a pain," he squinted.

"A pain, where exactly?" Clara tried to pinpoint the location and type of pain, but the patient explained that it hurt all throughout his lungs as he exhaled.

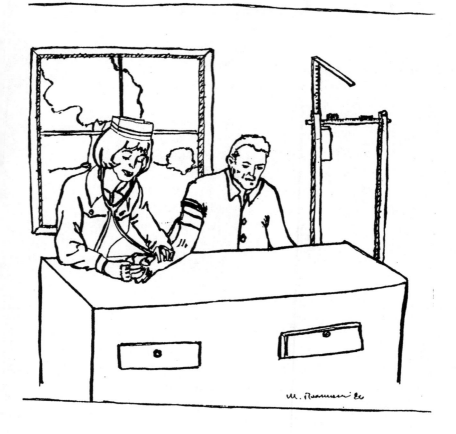

"Well, we'll let the doctor know that." Clara patted Mr. Druserenski on the back gently. "That's why you're here, to find out what's wrong and how we can help."

"Okay," he sighed and sat down, with a sad expression on his face. After Clara finished writing down a few things, she tried to reassure him, then excused herself. She returned a minute later.

"All right, just follow me right down here to room number three. Have a seat and Dr. Loy will be right in." Mr. Druserenski followed her and walked into the room.

"Thank you nurse."

"Well, I hope you start feeling better. Take care," Clara said as she walked back toward the sitting room to work up the next patient.

Max, a fourteen year old boy had been in gym class when an asthma attack occurred. Although he appeared to be only wheezing mildly at this time, it was obvious that he had just suffered an attack. He appeared upset and tired and sat with his fists on the chair so that he could brace himself as he leaned forward to get more comfortable. His mother looked extremely concerned. Clara escorted the two of them to the treatment room.

Two hours later, Clara looked at her watch, stepped around the corner to find out if any charts or people sat in the waiting room. She walked back, straightened up the two chairs and picked up a Kleenex off the floor and tossed it into the wastebasket. She took her calculator and put it in her pocket, then headed for the receptionist's desk.

"See you Monday, Andrea . Jo Ellen, say bye to Maria."

"See you later Clara." Andrea waved.

"Bye, have a nice weekend." Jo Ellen reached for the telephone and waved goodbye while Clara smiled back.

Then Clara sneezed and as she walked away, she heard her friends simultaneously say, "Gesundheit". She recalled a German friend from her childhood who informed her that the word actually is used to wish a person good health, not say "bless you," as she had assumed.

CHAPTER 10

"Henry," George nagged. "We have to discuss this, we're running out of time and a lot of the other reactors want to know if you're with us or not. Remember, pals, buddies, like we used to say. I can't figure out what's going on in that mind of yours, you agreed that you wouldn't sit by passively while the enemy attacked. Right?" prodded George.

"That's what I said, I suppose, but there's more to it than that, George, and I'm not sure I can make you or the rest of them understand."

"Understand what? For Pete's sake, if you tell me, I can let you know if I understand or not."

"George, it's not a simple matter. If I just had a little more time, maybe I could think of a way," I hedged.

But George got serious all of a sudden and emphasized that time kept ticking by and told me that I would have to tell him what was bothering me so that I could clear the air once and for all. "Tomorrow, Henry, that's it," he said to me. "I got word that all of the high risk factors will be in full swing. They're going to need us Henry."

"Okay George, I'll be there, but remember what you said about believing in my strategic mind and especially my experience. I want to plant that idea firmly in your head, because there may come a time when I need you to rely on the way I say to do things, even if it goes beyond some high-ranking superiors. Now I need to know if you're with me!" I looked dead into my friend's eyes.

"Well, can't say that I understand completely, but I'm registering what you tell me. I'm taking it to heart, Henry, okay pal? Will that do for now? Unless you want to elaborate," he coaxed.

"I think we've said enough for now. Let's go locate those two sources you have and do some digging and see if we can get any more information, what do you say?" I asked.

"All right. Let's go."

"This way, we'll go check with Vessel Police Force," directed George.

As we moved about in Clara's circulation, we discussed the old days and how much progress had been made in the area of understanding immunology and ways to prevent diseases.

"The plague, polio, typhoid fever, measles, mumps, rabies, viruses, those all used to be the killers," I pointed out.

"Yeah, nowadays, it's all sorts of different antigens, still have some deadly viruses, self-destructive lifestyles, and the AIDS epidemic that we have to fight. I've been hearing some strange things lately, as if we're regressing occasionally due to shortages of vaccines, and those unexpected over-reactive cases. There was a young boy in Georgia who became an invalid after his shots. It caused a panic, and before you knew it, the whole community, people all over the world, after the press got wind of it, didn't have any faith anymore in the immunization process. I don't know what the solution is there do you?" asked George.

"It's a tough one George, I don't know. It's a real dilemma. I've done some research on that though. Seems like we just have to protect against epidemics and yet for the one in a million or one in 300,000 that gets stuck with death or a permanent disability, it doesn't seem fair, the worst kind of tragedy happens," I rationalized.

"Say, did you ever wish you were human?" He asked me another question.

"What, and have to learn to adapt to that crazy world out there, no thanks. Those humans can be complicated creatures sometimes. Besides, I couldn't get used to the multi-shaded or shaven hairstyles or some of

the ridiculous crime rates. I'll stay put, right here inside
my little environment. At least in here I know what I'm up
against. That world scares me sometimes, but I think it
shows so much promise, you know, the American dream
and all that. I've seen it happen," I elaborated, "and the
people out there, well you know how terrific and good-
hearted some of them can be. I guess it's the old concept of
good versus evil that frightens or baffles me more than
anything," I rambled on.

Then George started to clue me in on what he heard
a professor at Yale say once at a lecture, and it made a lot
of sense. It dealt with the subject of fear.

The professor emphasized the profound notion that
people are never really free of the fear of something unless
the individual is also free of the fear associated with it. In
other words, he meant to say, that the perception of a threat
can be just as harmful as the real threat.

I thought about Sara's adaptation to smoke and her
victory over the fear and threat of what smoke might do to
her as far as causing an asthma attack, and the way she
managed to utilize relaxation techniques sometimes to
avoid panicking during her worst attacks.

"Hmm," I scratched my head. "I think Dr. Hansel's
work was profound yet simplistic, in a way. After all,
adapting is supposed to be a basic phenomenon of humans
as well as animals. Yeah, I've read all about Dr. Hansel's
and Dr. Brownie's theories and research on stress and
adaptation. Did you ever get to hear them speak?" I
asked.

"Yes, I did see Dr. Hansel once, a year before he
passed away, and believe me, it was fascinating. Went
with a medical technologist to a seminar convention one
day. She was scurrying around looking for answers,
fluctuating between more traditional treatment and the
more extreme ecologically based emphasis. God Henry,
what a day. You never would have believed it if you hadn't

seen it with your own eyes. All day Saturday, we sat through speaker after speaker, at this spectacular hotel in Reno. You're aware of the difference, right, between more conservative allergists and what they call clinical ecologists? And then the psychologists, some who lean toward physiological maladaptations, others who lean toward psychological origins in regards to disease states?"

"Yes George, what happened?" I asked excitedly. I listened in awe while my buddy talked about history being made that day. A big debate had taken place.

"Dr. Hansel was there, more as a mediator than anything else. Both sides had provided lectures and presented patients who had been treated by all different types of therapies. Some of them told the saddest stories. People who even moved out of their houses and searched for, or constructed, a less allergenic environment. And the angry ones, people who had been told over and over again, that it was all in their head, that their allergies or intolerances, their multitude of physiological responses didn't even exist. (That we, antibodies, didn't even exist or do our jobs.) Henry, it was pathetic at times."

I told him to continue.

"Anyway, philosophical mediators and Dr. Hansel were working throughout the day, and by dusk they had managed to bring about what seemed to be the impossible. Everyone, I mean everyone, was shaking hands. I don't know how they did it. All of the leftist psychologists shaking hands with the right winged ones. Can you imagine, Freudians and Jungian types merging? Immunologists shared information and kept an open ear to all of the various theories. Clinical psychologists and other allergists met in one room and debated hot issues. Everyone listened to the other side of the story, and agreed to merge forces, for the sake of the patients. Afterwards, there was an inspiring celebration. You should have seen their faces, the happiness, the peace, and relief. I felt as if I

was watching a post-war celebration. What a day,"
George took a deep breath, then sighed.

At this point, I felt utterly bewildered by George's
long, highly fabricated speech. I did, however, let him
finish before saying something about the way he always
managed to throw in his own happy ending tales, because I
truly liked George's "stories".

"Yeah, even the allergic victims themselves, they
promised to concentrate on all areas of health education:
good sound nutrition, adequate rest and relaxation, meds,
exercise, sexuality, emotional issues, and certain do's and
don'ts that allergic individuals have to pay attention to.
Also, adequate interests, purpose in life and social support."

"Social support?" I wanted him to elaborate.

"A medical sociologist said that boredom and
loneliness can be contributing factors in a person's illness
or ability to improve. And everyone at the convention
agreed on and emphasized the connection between the body
and mind, and the remarkable potential which people have
to help themselves toward an optimum point with
conscientious, persistent rehabilitative effort and support.
The allergic and asthmatic individuals vowed to work on
internal control as well as external circumstances," He
rambled on enthusiastically. "They explained that realistic
limitations may make it more difficult for some people, but
they acknowledged the fact that there was always an
optimal level of functioning to strive for."

"Say, George, uh buddy." He still looked like he
was daydreaming, actually reliving the event. (I thought to
myself, you sure can be a real Danny Kaye-Walter Mitty
character sometimes.) "You know, I sure don't recall
hearing anything about this historical, monumental
convention, and being an antibody you'd think I'd know if
something like this took place. Are you certain about this
unforgettable day in history, that it took place exactly like

you said?" I added a patronizing tone of voice, without meaning to.

George frowned and turned toward me with a shameful look on his face. "Ah Henry, I'm sorry. I got a little carried away again, didn't I? Well darn it, it doesn't hurt to dream, does it? I think we're all getting closer to answers and working together, it might happen someday. I'm sorry bud, for giving you all that fairy tale stuff. Why didn't you stop me, let me carry on that way, like an old fool? But the convention Henry, it happened, just not quite like I told it."

I empathized with him. "I know George, we all want to hope for the best. And they are getting to the bottom of things with better research and more understanding health care. Things will work out. It just takes awhile."

"I don't know," he said sadly, "sometimes I just wonder about it all, about my life, my job, you know? Last month I had to work on this transplant case, was lucky to escape with my old life. Well, you know how tricky it is with those transplant cases, you've endured some."

"Yeah, a few. I know how dangerous they are. You've had one recently huh? Did the person make it?" I asked, hoping the victim lived.

"Not this one, I'm afraid. I don't even know what I was doing there, since I'm an allergy specialist, but they transferred me anyway. Was a darn shame too. We fought like crazy for that little guy. Sometimes, I just...," he began to cry, but held back, "I uh, just wouldn't work another one of those, that's all I know. I'd quit first."

"Yeah, I know George, me too. How old?"

"Only six." George described the loss, how a bunch of phagos, macros and lymphos worked with the antibody troops. But the little boy, Berry, died anyway. Later, some high-rankers that weren't even at the death scene, but had given the orders then escaped, were to be court-martialed.

The charges were poor judgment. They pleaded 'rejection phenomenon' and got off. But there were a lot of education classes after that, all concerning over-reaction, personal liability, and how nobody can ever escape it. All of the transplant specialists had to take the classes. Recommended them for everyone else too."

"I heard about this George, except that you were involved. I didn't know you were there. It must have been a close call then, hmm?"

"Believe me, it was. There were only a few of us that reached the conclusion in time, that we had to retreat or die, that's what it came down to Henry. We couldn't persuade the others, so we waited for a blood transfusion one day and got out by passive transfer. Henry, it just wasn't my time to go yet. I felt like a real coward that day. But I wish it could have been different. I wish it with all my heart. In a sense, I guess, I felt somewhat of a rebel too, knowing the truth of the matter, not willing to follow the old train of thought."

"There weren't any survivors left, were there?" I asked.

"No, not the ones who stayed. It was one of those cases that meant victory or all out defeat for everyone. We all lost that day. A sad day in history."

I thought to myself, maybe it's not going to be so hard to make George understand after all. My friend was feeling a great deal of pain, but I didn't really know what to say, so I didn't say anything. After that conversation though, I felt relieved and more comfortable around him. Some of the anxiety had disappeared.

"Here he is, Vessel Patrol Officer Geno. Geno, how's it going, busy tonight?" George switched moods and smiled.

"A little more than usual, not too bad. George, what are you up to?" The patrolbody tipped his hat.

"I need to find Richy and Porter, you know where they are? This is a friend of mine, Henry, he's new on this case." He introduced us.

"Hi. Pleasure."

"Hi." I smiled and offered my hand.

"Well, Richy's out on pollen grain watch and Porter's on dog dander duty. Always a little action there." Geno stuck his hands in his pockets.

"What time are they reporting in?"

"At 2200 hours," Geno said.

"Okay, listen, will you tell them George wants to talk to them, to stop by the cell tonight, nothing important. Just want to ask them something."

"Sure will. Are you sure you don't want me to leave a message of any sort?" Geno coaxed.

"No, I just want to ask them about switching one day next week with Henry and myself. Thanks. See you later," said George.

"Hey George, do you think he'd know anything?"

" I wouldn't want to ask him. They say he reports everything. I mean everything and anything out of the ordinary. I don't trust the guy. He's too much like a robot. Think he's trying to brown-nose his way up to commander."

"Hmm. Great." I answered sarcastically.

At 10:30 p.m. sharp, there was a knock at George's membrane. He found out what he wanted to know, but couldn't figure out what the exact danger was yet. Clara planned to go camping over the weekend with her husband. They mentioned horseback riding in a conversation last week. That's the only thing George could think of. He remembered her allergic reactions before, on other rides. Richy and Porter were to keep their ears open. He said goodnight and then we all decided to get some rest.

"We'll talk to Major Magen tomorrow. He lives right next door. He's a good one to talk to," George explained as I stood at his cell door.

"Okay George, you know the situation around here better than I do."

We both retired and I fell asleep within the half hour after trying to figure out what the danger might be. My eyes were closed, but I kept trying to piece things together and thought about George's ordeal and comments that he had made today. I knew we were on the same wavelength now, whereas, before, I wasn't certain.

CHAPTER 11

Early in the morning, the Major heard a knock at his membrane.

"George, I'm glad you're here. I've got to clue you in on some things." Major Magen welcomed us.

"How much time is left before we know what the source of the problem is?" asked George.

"Well, we won't know until it hits her, but we've narrowed down the possibilities. "Hi," he turned toward me. "Who's your friend, George?"

"Oh, this is Henry. Henry, Major Magen. He's with us all the way, Sir." George glanced at me with a piercing look.

"Hello, Major Magen, nice to meet you." I smiled and offered my hand.

"So, you're going to give us some extra help, well, we're probably going to need you. Glad you're here. Now let's sit down. Like I was saying, the foreigners we'll be looking for are pollen, mold, etc. She's been overdosing on some of her favorite foods too, so watch that. The digestive reactors have battled it out the last day or so due to a large milk shake. The monthly hormonal shifts are causing the reactors to behave hypersensitively. Also, keep an eye out for insect, bee or snake bites. That's a possibility since she's planning a hike in the foothills. It's rare, but it could happen. Other than that, perhaps the exercise-induced problem, but that's usually controlled by her inhalers."

The Major then explained that he would spend the next couple of hours preparing the regiments, assigning posts and informing the troops about the anticipation of a severe reaction. He made it clear, without prompting from either George or myself, that no fighting or explosive reactions were appropriate unless he gave the orders.

He said very seriously to us, "Remember, this is a Code Red Emergency Alert. They've got to be ready. Expect orders from Sergeant Birlly, myself, or their commanders on duty. Oh, the IGE battalion, they'll have orders to stay at their posts and wait, because if the antigens come right to them, no need to advance. Captain Kale will be there to give the explosive orders. George, make sure we have a stocked supply of granules ready. She's leaving about 0900 hours. That gives us at least three hours to have everyone man their battle stations. It's up to us to protect her." He looked dead at us. "Henry, George, may God be with us."

"Yes Sir," George said. I saluted and said the same. "We're on our way Sir."

I paused on my way out, wanted to ask the Major something, but felt a nudge from George and changed my mind.

"We'll be ready for whatever it is. We all want to save her, right Sir?" George risked prolonging our stay and emphasizing the issue I wanted to stress, saving the girl rather than destroying her.

"Absolutely. Now, I'm headed over to the T and B regiments, I've got to make sure they're standing by. I'll get back to you later, let's say ten-hundred hours."

George grabbed my arm and we hurriedly began to organize Clara's self defense troops.

CHAPTER 12

"What a beautiful morning. It's just perfect. Bret, wake up." Clara nudged her husband, but he failed to respond, except to twitch his right foot. Clara stepped out of bed, opened the front door, glanced at the sky and took a few deep breaths. The cool morning air filled her nostrils. She noticed the clear sky, the quietness, and watched the sparrows bathing in the birdbath while some of them scrounged around the ground for food particles. While bending over to pick up the newspaper, she read the headlines.

"SURGEON COMES FORWARD AFTER TWENTY-NINE YEARS. HIS BOOK, JFK (CONSPIRACY OF SILENCE) REVEALS ASTOUNDING FACTS."

After turning off the porch light, she walked to the kitchen and tossed the paper on the table.

"Honey." She walked into the bedroom. "Time to get up. Remember, you said we'd leave by nine or so." Bret groaned and turned over on his right side.

"I'll fix up some scrambled eggs and toast. You have to wake up, or it'll be the cold wash rag treatment," she threatened.

He opened his eyes widely. "I think it's about time we got going, don't you sweetheart? I'll go jump in the shower. Do you think I need to shave?"

Clara laughed at his abrupt alertness. "It's amazing how you wake up so fast sometimes. Shave? Let me feel your whiskers." She sat on the side of the bed, placed her right hand on his cheek and rubbed her palm against his face. He put his arms around her and kissed her. Clara nestled back down next to him. They embraced and began to childishly wrestle with each other.

"Bret! Bret! Stop, you're tickling me." Clara tried to make him stop.

"Hmm?" He kissed her neck, just below the left earlobe.

"Don't shave. I like your whiskers."

"And I like you. In fact, I love you."

"Oh I love you so much. I can never say it enough." After breakfast, Clara tried, discreetly, to hurry Bret along, so they could leave for the anticipated weekend adventure.

"Hey, by the way," Clara said, "You're supposed to cuddle with me under the stars tonight, not today in an ordinary bed. Remember? A bottle of lemonade and the 'sky as our ceiling'."

"Who said I forgot? I'll get the lemonade out of the refrigerator right now." He walked toward the kitchen. "I'll get the cheese spread and crackers now too." He yelled, "Are you ready for a good long hike, honey?"

"Yeah, I'm ready. Do you think we'll see any deer? Roy and Val," she shouted, "were up there a couple of weeks ago, not that park, but one close by and they saw some Mule deer. I asked them to go, but Val had a wedding to go to. Besides, it will be fun with just us."

As he finished up packing a few more items from the kitchen he headed for the bedroom. "I don't know, we could see some deer," he answered. "Did you decide yet on the horseback riding or not?"

"I think I want to go Bret, if you do. I'll take my medicine along, and if I sneeze, I'll just sneeze it out. I've got plenty of tissues and antihistamines, and my inhalers of course. Oh, and the anaphylactic kit, it's in the first aid pack."

Clara fed her dog Harvey. Julien, a friend, agreed to look after him for the weekend. One last pet by his masters and Bret and Clara were in the jeep driving toward Golden. Clara searched the map in her hand for Pine exit.

Once they found it, they could follow that road into Roundup State Park.

"Hey, it says here that the park 'is noted for a wide variety of wildlife, including deer, bear, mountain lion and wild turkey.' I'd love to see a lion." She continued to read. "Hiking/equestrian trails have been located on the perimeter of major wildlife habitat areas so as to allow the public to view the animals in their natural setting, yet not to disturb them. Therefore, it is of prime importance for the park user to stay on the trails that are provided. The park user should also be aware..." She stopped suddenly and read silently, then blurted out, "Listen to this, 'the park user should also be aware that the Diamond Back rattlesnake is found throughout the park, so caution should be exercised during the warm season'."

"You saw one before up here, didn't you?"

"Yeah, remember, I told you about it. I heard it. It was off the trail directly to the left of where I stepped. I looked and didn't see anything, but we ran out of there. You should have seen how scared Greg was. Remember, that day I went with Greg and June last year?"

"I remember. But you didn't see anymore after that or hear any?"

"No, that was it."

"What did the rattle sound like?"

"Just like a rattle. Like someone shaking a baby's rattle, maybe a little faster than usual," she explained.

"Hmm. There it is, Pine Road."

"I see it. It's a perfect day, too. Let me get the suntan lotion. It's warm already." She reached in the glove compartment and found a small tube of Coppertone and her make-up bag with her medicine inside. "Is the first aid kit still in the trunk?"

Bret decided to park under a shady tree. Clara grabbed items from the back seat as he unloaded the trunk. He scattered everything on the ground. Off to the left, the

first aid kit caught his eye. He told Clara to stick it in her
backpack.

"It's great having my very own EMT around. This
kit has everything. You really stuffed it." After some
organizing, and changing into hiking shoes, the two of
them began to hike along the sloped dirt trail. Bret held a
map in his hand that designated which direction to follow
in order to find the camping area. The bright sun and dry
air was refreshing. Clara thought to herself, finally, we're
here. "God I love the outdoors. It's so beautiful and
peaceful." He shared his wife's exact thoughts.

CHAPTER 13

"It's windy today, huh. I hate windy days," Clara said.
"Why?"
"I don't know, unless I'm flying a kite, I just never liked the wind. I can't seem to think straight in it, and it makes my ears hurt." She stopped and let the backpack slide down off of her shoulders. "Here, wait sweety, I'm going to put some Kleenex in them, let's stop for just a second."

"Nag, nag, nag." Bret said facetiously.

Clara, on the other hand, took his comments seriously. "I'm not nagging, just telling you something, there's a difference." After tearing off a small piece of tissue, she formed two little round balls and inserted them in each ear. "There, that's better."

"All set?" He hoisted her blue backpack up over her shoulders.

"Know what?" Clara said.

"What?"

"I keep thinking about the movie last night. The last part was pretty tough to digest, wasn't it?"

"What do you mean?"

"Well, it was such a parallel. There's her boyfriend, so happy, calling to tell her that they finally got Carnegie Hall, the first time for a jazz singer, a dream come true. And there she is, hugging the dead and bloody piano man. All because she had to go and get messed up again. It was so tragic."

"Yeah, I wonder what happened next, but I guess we'll never know, since a certain person had to get up and turn the TV off." He tried to swat a fly that had landed on his left arm.

"Well, I'm sorry, but I just couldn't watch it anymore. They always do that. It couldn't end happily.

She should have made it. (What's with all these flying, hopping grasshoppers? She mumbled to herself.) I know that they had to depict reality. Drug addiction is a tough thing to beat and I guess Billie Holiday was just one of the unlucky ones. It's a shame, so many lives are ruined, so many broken dreams, just because some people have to abuse drugs and alcohol."

"Well, you know better than anyone else, Clara, with your mom."

"I know. It hurts so bad sometimes. I wish she could have a different kind of life, a healthy life. She's so beautiful in so many ways. And yet, we have to watch her head down a dead-end street." They hiked along the trail, silent for a few minutes.

"Here, let's go to the right here." Bret pointed.

"Okay, you're the leader."

They both made an angular turn and continued hiking up a trail called Wild Arrow. "But you know what, I think I understand alcoholism a lot better these days. How it just ruined aspects of my mom's life." Her words sounded choppy. She took a deep breath and huffed and puffed while climbing as the slope steepened.

"Well, you know you don't have to tell me, the AA veteran."

Clara smiled and took another deep breath. "You know, if you think about it, some of the nicest people around, the most sensitive, creative or famous, or even prominent people in the world are alcoholics or past alcoholics. The thing I always worried most about was my parents drinking and driving. Why is it that when someone is hurting or heading toward self-destruction, they refuse to get help and work toward getting better? I want her to get well, to stop drinking so much and stop smoking herself to death. Can I sit down just for a second, okay?" Feeling exhausted, Clara noticed a large rock and headed for it.

Bret teased, "Can't talk and walk at the same time, you know what they say."

"I know, I know. I wish I had the money. I'd send her to one of those fancy health resorts or well-known rehabilitation centers, or I guess if she'd just go to AA. And now she's coughing so much with that evil cancer. Poor mom. She's always sick. I always wished for some magic power so I could give her better health, a better life."

"I like your mom too, a lot, but I hate to see her like this." He shook his head from side to side.

Clara became pensive, visions of last month when her mom had adverse reactions to some drugs haunted her. She had found her mom sleepy and sick, mumbling about taking some pills. Scared, but not panicky, Clara dialed 911 and the dispatcher told her he would send an ambulance right away. Clara realized later, that her mom would have died if she had not found her in time.

Attempting to sound positive, Clara said, "But Mom's been trying to cut down on her drinking. I just spoke to her the other day and she's eating a little better, orders by her doctor."

"Good. Hey, how come your dad can handle his drinking without getting sick?"

"I don't know. He just does. I think it's because he eats better than mom and gets some nutrition, mostly home cooking, whereas mom seems to eat just sandwiches and supper once and awhile. And I think, you know, the male versus female way of life, mom worries about everything and dad just says 'such is life' and takes things in stride."

"Hmm. That sounds like your dad."

"Now, let's talk about our hiking trip!" Clara said excitedly.

"I'm all for that."

"We're going to hike up to the camping area, right?"

"Right!" Bret affirmed.

"Then get set up for the night, right?"

"Right!"

"Then go over to the stables right, and ride a horse."

"We'll try anyway, it's been awhile you know, and if you're sure you won't get sick on me."

"Then what?" asked Clara.

"I don't know," he paused. "Maybe walk some more, or get out the grill and cook supper, or the Scrabble game or cards and see if you can beat me. And then get ready for our bottle of lemonade and night under the stars."

"Sounds romantic to me. Will you really play Scrabble? Usually, I have to beg you."

"Yeah, if we're not too tired from everything else, sure."

"Okay. All it takes is a little mind power anyway and enough energy to pick up the letters." Clara's wheezing got louder.

"You sound like you're having troubles."

"Yeah, I need to spray. I can't walk and talk at the same time, and this altitude isn't helping." Clara reached into her pockets for her blue inhaler device and tiny bottle of eye drops. After shaking the inhaler and exhaling, simultaneously, she put her lips around the opening and inhaled as she pressed down. She soon took a second puff.

After a brief rest, they hiked past a sign posted on a fence to their right which read, "RIFLE RANGE: KEEP OUT". Downtown Denver and three small manmade lakes were clearly visible as they reached the peak of a vista point.

After passing another sign which pointed toward GABLE'S STABLES, Clara stepped quickly to the left to avoid a pile of dried up horse manure. The dirt trail became sandy, then rocky again, and zigzagged in a north and south direction, mostly sloping upward, but occasionally easing with a brief downhill slope. A quiet mood fell upon Clara and Bret as the wind made the pine trees sway. The only sounds were a few buzzing bees, and several birds chirping in the distance. They hiked another three-fourths of a mile and had to decide which trail to take.

"According to this, we can take Hayride, the long way around, or turn right toward the campsite with Indianhead. What do you think, walk straight to it, save time so we can go horseback riding?"

"Sure," agreed Bret, "that sounds good."

It was only another half a mile until they reached the campsite. The temperature exceeded ninety degrees, and the perspiration dropped off of their faces as they hiked and stopped occasionally to sip cold water from a yellow picnic jug. Suddenly, Bret stopped and pointed, trying to get Clara's attention, but she kept looking down at her feet while walking until she almost bumped into him as he stood perfectly still.

"There. Look," he whispered and stared at a very large gray deer off in the distance. The deer stood motionless and stared back.

"Oh, how gorgeous. He's so neat." Clara whispered. "Look at him look right at us, like wanting to ask us what the heck we're doing here."

"Well, this is his territory." They both admired the wild animal for a few more moments, then hiked until they reached a sign with an arrow on it, designating that the campsite veered directly to the left. A green water pump off to the right also caught their attention.

"Look, we have extra water! Let's go try it." Excitedly they neared the water pump, but then both of them were startled by a hornet that kept whizzing by. Clara screamed the first time it flew by her.

"Clara, don't scream! It will just attract its' attention."

"I know. But it scares me." She began to walk backward away from the pump. "You get the water. I'm going to check out the campsite. Be careful." She ran toward a grassy area and yelled, "Bye."

Bret proceeded calmly, but cautiously, ignoring the bee. He placed both hands on the long slender handle and pushed it downward and pulled it back up again, until the water gushed out from the green pump. After dropping his backpack to the ground, he searched for a small pink picnic jug. He filled the jug to the top, tasted the water, which was quite cold. Then he walked over to the campsite where Clara had already made herself at home.

"Did you have any bee problems?"

"Nope. No problems. I think the little rascal was gone." He set his backpack down. "Hey, this is nice here, huh?"

"It's beautiful, all this open space, I love it."

He noticed the beauty and solitude of the location. They were surrounded by a few trees, and grassy open areas to the east and north of them. Several pieces of driftwood had been skillfully placed around a grill.

"They even have a grill ready for us, and some driftwood to sit on. This is perfect. Looks like someone was here just recently."

"Sure does, doesn't it. Maybe yesterday." He walked over to Clara and sat next to her. He hugged her and she wrapped her arms around him. They kissed several times. Then he asked, "Are you going to help me set up the tent?"

"Sure." But neither one of them moved. After another long kiss, Bret smiled and began to stare into Clara's ocean-blue eyes.

"You know what?"

"What?" Clara wondered if something romantic was coming.

"I could remain lost forever in these mountains with you."

"Me too. God I love you." She kissed him passionately again. "No wait. The idea would be, to be found forever, and together, not lost," Clara said seriously.

He laughed, "Okay, okay. Found then, and together. Let's get this tent set up."

CHAPTER 14

"Major! Major! We heard Geno yell as he pounded on Major Magen's membrane. He responded immediately. Geno explained, "I've sounded the alarms, Sir, this could be it, foreigners have been spotted in the bloodstream! She's on a horse right now!"

"Foolish woman. I knew she'd have trouble with that horse idea. What the heck's she waiting for? Why doesn't she take her medicine? Give orders to react, but only accordingly, with reasonable due progression. Any doubts or concerns, get back to me first. Geno, tell George and Henry to get up to those nasal and bronchus lines, to help wherever they can. And Geno, keep watch for Code Red Emergency Status. We're going to prevent or combat against any critical ordeals here. I like this little lady, understand?" His voice was gruff and commanding.

"Yes Sir! Got it Sir!" He saluted. Next, Geno pounded on our membrane. We all saluted each other and prepared ourselves mentally for battle.

Here's a little secret I'll share with you. The weakness in our immune army stems from the fact that we're always playing defense in these wars, never making the first preventive move. We can't, because we're reactors, counter attackers. Once the barrier is broken and the plasma cells fire the signal, only then do we act and then we overdue it.

George and I circulated up to the swollen bronchial tubes as ordered. We overheard the sinister intruders. The creeps were boasting about how they infiltrated. Most of them sifted through the nasal membranes, others by mouth. Keep in mind, this was just one location in the body, they were probably everywhere by now.

One little sneak started jabbing at one of Clara's cell membranes. "Hey, Vernie, Charlie, Tobie, Kristie, c'mon.

Dig in! Let's go, this is what we're here for! The Sarge and Major aren't around. I'm not waitin' for any orders. They'd want us to tear into her anyway."

At that moment, George and I gritted our teeth and watched from a distance as our surface antibodies decided they had taken enough from the heartless enemies, and it was time to react.

"Neutralize!" One of our commanders ordered.

"Kill! Kill!" The antigen named Vernie yelled.

I found myself shouting back orders too, so we could counter-attack and neutralize, as I lunged out at one of the antibodies. George was directly behind me cursing the relentless little creatures and charging too. We were holding our own when a skinny, mean antigen conked us on the head.

"Hon," Clara blinked her itching, red, swollen eyes and sniffled constantly as she spoke. "I've got to stop for a minute. Whoa, Wildfire, Whoa." The chocolate brown horse listened to her command, slowed down, and came to a halt. Bret turned his head, just for a second, but realized he was very close to a barbed wire fence to the right, so he looked straight ahead and guided the horse to the left, until he could stop. "What's the matter?" he shouted.

"What do you mean, what's the matter, the usual," Clara said sarcastically, but not loud enough for him to hear. "I'm having a sneezing, wheezing fit. Can't breathe and my eyes are killing me. I need water and my medicine."

"Geez, look at your right eye, it's almost swollen shut Clara." Bret held onto his horse, dismounted, then walked back to Clara. "Here, hold onto these, I'll get the water out. Didn't you take something before we left? My God, you should see your eyes." He hurried to find the jug.

"Wait a second. I, I can't talk right now." She put the reigns in one hand and reached into her pocket for her inhaler. She went through the process, very quickly, of

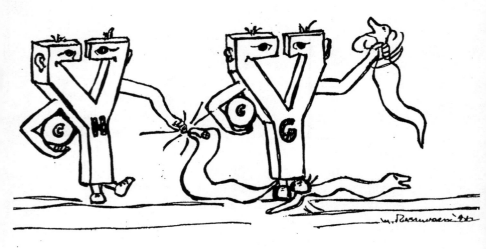

administering a dose of medication. She tried to attend to the horses who were quiet but restless. However, she couldn't see very well, due to the condition of her eyes.

"Here." He handed her the water and grabbed the reins. "Now, what do you have to take, an antihistamine?"

"Yeah. And my eye drops. This makes me so mad!" She sipped some water and swallowed an antihistamine capsule. "Guess I messed up. I thought maybe I wouldn't have that much trouble if I wore gloves and used just the one inhaler. Obviously, I was wrong." She blew her nose several times on a tissue she had found.

Next, she proceeded to place two drops of liquid medicine into her eyes to reduce the itching and redness.

She apologized again. "Sorry about this. But you know what, at least it goes away about as fast as it comes on. I hope. That's what happened anyway, a couple of years ago when I went riding with Liz and her cousin Eva. I didn't even take anything that day. It just acted up, then subsided about an hour after I got off the horse."

"Yeah, well, it might settle down. But apparently today, you needed that antihistamine," he said seriously. "You couldn't have some kind of curable illness, you have to have allergies."

"Well, excuse me. I didn't pick my health problem. I cannot help it if I have wild and crazy antibodies wandering around in my body," Clara responded.

"Are you ready to go now?"

"I'm ready."

"Did you hear that, Henry, she called us wild and crazy."

"Yeah, yeah, I heard. Oh my aching head. How long have we been out?" He rubbed the back of his head.

"I don't know for sure. Long enough evidently. Everything looks calm again. Let's check out the damage and report back to the Major."

67

"Maybe that was it ,George, what do you think, the big scare?"

"Don't know Henry, we'll have to wait and see."

"Yeah, we sure don't want to take any chances, be left off guard," his buddy agreed.

Bret helped position Clara's backpack and asked if she wanted to head back.

"No. I want to follow the trail around. I'll be all right. I'll probably get a little sleepy later with this pill though. Okay, let's go." She steadied herself on the horse as she fitted herself into the stirrups.

"Sure, if you're ready. Can you see now?"

"Yes. My left eye's fine. The other one will get better soon."

"Well, be careful."

"I will. If I have to stop for something, I'll say so, but I should be all right now." She tried to reassure him.

"Hi-Ho Silver, and a way we go," he joked. Clara and Bret both laughed as they rode along. After the horseback ride, they hiked back to their campsite.

CHAPTER 15

" Let's just sit here for a little while. It's so peaceful."
Clara straightened out her sleeping bag and laid it
on the ground. "I knew I'd get sleepy with that pill
I took. Gosh, I can't believe we did it, rode a horse. Can
you?"

"Yeah I can believe it all right, even feel it. In fact,
at this moment my rear-end is reminding me of the bumpy
ride. Seems to me it didn't ache this much back when I was
a kid and rode with my brothers." He snuggled up next to
Clara and put his arm around her.

"Hey, do you think our lives are too fast-paced?"
she asked, then added, "I mean, don't you ever wonder
about living a different kind of life?

"Well, sure I do. Sometimes I think about all of the
different kinds of lives, occupations in the world. You
know, upper class, us stuck in the middle class, people
who live in poverty, maybe living somewhere else, maybe
on a ranch, or running our own business or something. you
know, stuff like that. What about you, hon?"

After a few seconds of thought, Clara answered
assuredly, "I'd be a musician, or writer, someone who never
gives up on that inner voice, or motivation to follow that
musical or creative unique quality about myself. Know
what I mean?"

He took a sip of water from the jug then offered it to
Clara. "I know what you mean, exactly." He mentioned
how the creative ones usually live painful lives, though,
kind of a roller-coaster existence, but figure it's worth it. "I
don't know how they do it. Then there's the talented young
baseball player, or say great piano player who is persuaded
by parents or friends or orthodox schooling to get into
something more lucrative, some unsuitable trade. You've
talked about this before, how sometimes creativity or things
people have a passion for are given consideration last."

"Yeah. It's like telling someone to give up their dreams. I realize you can't live off of dreams entirely, but we sure need our dreams and goals too, especially in this world. I think people do have to be careful though. Dreams are okay, but only if someone perseveres and does the foundation work necessary to make them come true." Clara reached for his hand.

"Exactly. That's why I have to start that paramedic course and my photography again, too. I haven't taken any pictures in about six months. This teaching job for the Red Cross is rewarding, but it's not enough. I'm beginning to feel like I'm in too much of a routine, too unchallenged. I need something to break that."

"Your dark room's waiting for you right downstairs." Clara smiled. "And you'll be buried in medical books pretty soon. The holidays are coming up in a few months, let's make a pact to do something over Thanksgiving and Christmas. I'll get back to my poetry and you can work on taking some unique photos and your studies."

He glanced at his wristwatch and realized it was time to get started with dinner. "What do you think about some dinner? We've had good conversation, now let's have some appetizing food." He sat up. "What do you think?"

"I think I'll be waiting for an artistic photo for the living room, and yes, I'm hungry. What do we need? Matches, water. What else?" They both helped each other to a standing position. Bret rubbed his butt and moaned while Clara laughed about it. Then she kissed him on the cheek.

He decided to dig out the pans, dishes and other stuff from his backpack while Clara found the matches and set the small cooler of food near the campfire site.

"Great," Bret said as Clara handed him the matches. "I'll see if I can get what I need and get this thing started.

Will you run and get some water? I rinsed out my stinky shirt with that other and this one's almost empty too."

"Sure." She picked up the jug.

"Be careful," he reminded her due to the incident with the bee earlier.

He rearranged the ashy, remaining logs and pile of thinner kindling they had gathered. He placed a firestarter log and some newspaper in the center and with the first match was successful. A few of the stones had gotten displaced, outside the circle, so he carefully replaced them to contain the fire. He dug out the battery operated tape player and decided to set the outdoor mood with some Fleetwood Mac. He thought about Bruce Springsteen or Mellancamp, but changed his mind, considering the serene, Rocky Mountain nature setting. Just like fishing, he thought to himself, don't want to disturb or scare away the wild animals. "Like I said ," he mumbled, "it's their home, not ours."

CHAPTER 16

The next thing you're going to learn about old Henry here, is that I'm tired. Tired of fightin' it, tired of trying to break through the iron wall of skepticism. I won't deny that some humans, not the majority, may use allergies as a wastebasket diagnosis, occasionally, for their multitude of physical, psycho-social, and spiritual problems. And I wouldn't be surprised if somewhere along the line, the plea of an allergic disease has been or will be used as a scapegoat, to excuse some type of criminal behavior.

The point I'm trying diligently and honestly to make, by telling my story, is that there are millions, literally millions, of legitimate allergy and asthma stricken people out there. In fact, more asthmatics than ever before are dying each year, because of poor education or management of their very real killer disease.

Now it's true with allergies, there's not always an immune connection. Sometimes it is actually an intolerance or an idiosyncrasy of some sort toward specific irritants or substances, or say the asthmatic system's reaction to proteins or inefficient enzymes, just some of the things I kept trying to get across, like over-reacting to harmless things, but nobody would listen.

But believe me, they're out there, struggling along. I'm talking about the bodies that go haywire day after day, the uncontrolled cases, the disagreeable kid who's doped up with the meds by age six, and still feels like a zombie. There's the child who lies down on the floor and starts kicking and crying five minutes after eating a banana or some peanuts. That describes Arnie, another case, a bright, but tortured little boy. I worked with him for years. Finally his mom and dad took him to a board certified allergist. With his allergies managed, he became a healthy, thriving youngster, and his future was saved. Same thing with that other kid, you know, that miracle dust mite case.

I'd like to see a person who thinks allergies or asthma is nothing but a figment of a weak imagination, explain the deaths of people I've worked with, like Marin, or the ones I've heard or read about, horrible, sad, unnecessary deaths.

People who died frightening, tragic deaths because of their allergic or asthmatic nature, cases that involved infants and two year olds, teenagers and adults. The skeptic can work my job for awhile, any day. I wish I could be human just for a day, or if I figure out some miracle of a way to get my story into the hands of humans, I'd say, "Look, here I am. My name is Henry, and I'm very real. What does real mean? It means I exist. And if I exist, then my negative parallel also exists, the relentless antigen. Yes sir, I'd say, I'm an antibody and there really is a war going on inside hypersensitive individuals." Then, I'd show them a video of some of the wars, as well as casualties, that have occurred. I'd convince them, once and for all. Even some of the expert psychologists who damaged victims further by professing that someone should have total control over their health, their fates.

Sometimes, when victims died, overuse of medication, or the lack of it caused the final outcome. But so often, no matter how much sincere effort and emergency medical attention the unfortunate patient received after the fact, it was too late, the body was already too far gone, and just wouldn't respond. Same thing with all of the anaphylactic cases, like Marin and Clara, almost. Those darn, rotten allergies. I don't want to burn anybody's ears with a four letter or six letter word but that's how I feel.

And I'm well aware that the individual has a responsibility to do all he/she can to keep the body's resistance level at a maximum. They can tell me that humans have emotions that tie in, I can buy that. But how is an infant, or a two or four year or ten year old going to have such a tough time with emotions, that it causes such a fatal, immune reaction? It makes me sick to think about the misconceptions regarding allergies and asthma, and the warmongers, my own species, the ones who won't pull back before it's too late.

If there's one thing I've learned, because of Clara and Marin especially, it's the realization that at some point in time, an antibody must stop merely reacting and take fate into his or her own hands. That's where I do believe in the possibility of control. When education is maximized and understanding is accurate, and when everything possible is being done to prevent unnecessary, out of control, suffering; that's the high point I'd like to see the human race achieve, as well as antigens and antibodies.

In hindsight, the only thing that really could have saved Marin is some sort of preventative measures or an Adrenaline kit on hand, like Clara had. The saddest part about this a story is that so much of the misery and damage caused by allergies and asthma can be prevented by simply implementing health education and increasing understanding in these areas.

I've seen the agony that the antigen/antibody wars cause, I've tried to fight it, but I think I really need a break. I guess you could say I'm an antibody with limitations. One night last week, I sat wondering if the ones who do die are actually the lucky ones, because the long-lasting physical and mental torture that many of the living ones are subject to, frankly, just doesn't seem like it's worth it. Think about it. Doesn't the quality of a person's life mean anything? Especially the crippled ones, or the ones who have lost all signs of hope, or in essence, the ones who are physically here, but have died a thousand or more humiliating or emotional deaths. Probably even came close to physical death many times.

But I abandoned the dismal notion almost as quickly as I thought of it, because deep down I happen to be one of those eternal optimists. Where there's a living, breathing, albeit struggling, human being, there's hope. I've seen enough courageous survivors on respirators to know this. That means that I'm somebody who could never forsake the idea of hope.

But then I have friends who tell me never say never, because nobody knows what will happen in a lifetime. That always gets me to thinking about the what ifs, since I have witnessed a lot of human suffering, not to mention the anguish amidst my fellow antibodies.

So I decided to hang onto the notion that if I ever do feel sort of fatalistically tired, then I can still hang onto hope. The hope that ultimately good forces, rather than evil and positive solutions rather than negative ones will empower me to defy my darkest days the wrong to claim "victory".

CHAPTER 17

You're probably anxious to hear what happened to Clara. She did live. But believe me, she was only a matter of seconds from joining all of the other statistics. Just a few allergy facts first.

Individuals allergic to stings of Hymenopterous insects (bees, wasps, etc.) must be treated immediately to prevent a possible fatal outcome. The end can come very suddenly. In most cases, it happens within less than an hour, sometimes within minutes. Bee venom has immediate histaminic effects, but luckily, thank God, Clara and Bret were educated and conscientious enough to have an emergency kit on hand for the treatment of allergic reactions.

It took the quick-acting injection of Epinephrine to stabilize her until the Flight for Life helicopter arrived and the flight nurse and paramedic took over. They administered high flow oxygen with a non-rebreather mask. Luckily, the laryngeal edema was under control, so a tracheotomy was avoided. That's when they have to cut into the trachea (windpipe) without delay, to keep the victim breathing.

Bret performed well, as usual, in an emergency situation and simply did whatever he could and had to do, reflexively. But never before had he been so frightened, or witnessed the consequences of anaphylactic shock, a deadly allergic reaction which was about to kill his wife.

George, Major Magen, Richy, Porter, Sergeant Birlly, myself, and quite a few of the others, including two apologetic antigen converts, Sandy and Konnie; we all realized what was going on. The same old thing again, we couldn't get the rest of them to pull back after things were under control. Of course, they refused to listen. Once the lead attackers, Captain Gemly and Corporeal Skidder, broke through the border defenses, most of our reactors just went berserk. Tried to keep the inside perimeter intact, the outside from infiltrating, but fights broke out everywhere. Clara's whole body immediately turned into a battlefield, all out war with some of the Neutrophils attacking, once the command was given. And then it went on and on until they began to go crazy attacking everything in sight, including many of Clara's own cells.

George and I said our good-byes, got things off our chest, and did what any antibody in that predicament does, prepared to die. But converts and Bret saved us and Clara. Thank God. I think I'm the one who's in shock right now.

To the best of my recollection, it happened like this. The mood that afternoon at the campsite was one of serenity and light-heartedness. The smell of barbecued burgers still lingers upon my memory, like a lot of other things that day. The way Bret and Clara joked with each other until they both had side-aches from laughing so hard, then how their mood shifted suddenly to a sentimental one.

We sat in the shade and felt the most comforting breeze, and the quietness of the outdoors. You know, the kind of day that you wish would last forever. They were ready to taste their barbecued dinner when tragedy struck. I remember Bret saying, "Wait for me, wait for me."

"I'm waiting sweetheart, but it's all ready, c'mon, let's eat." Clara gestured with her hands.

"Okay, almost ready, just let me get the salt out of my backpack." He hurried over toward his gear.

When Clara reached out to pick up a can of grape soda, she heard a loud buzzing sound. It startled her. Jumping backward, she looked around and saw a bee on the ground where a piece of fruit had fallen earlier. Quickly, Clara grabbed her soda. As soon as she made contact, she felt a sharp stinging sensation to her right index finger, looked over, saw a yellow jacket, and screamed. "Bret, help!" she yelled desperately. "I've been stung." That's when Bret proceeded to save our lives.

"Oh God, a bee. What happened? Where's the kit?" Clara recognized the fear and sense of urgency which Bret displayed.

"In my backpack. Hurry Bret! I'm scared." She lifted her index finger to show him the sting.

"Oh no. It's red already and swelling. We know what to do, Clara. Don't worry. I'll get the injection." Then he looked at Clara and his controlled demeanor turned to fear. Her color had changed, and she wheezed and gasped for air. Bret grabbed her shoulders and tried to assist her to a more comfortable sitting position against the tree with the picnic blanket behind her back.

But Clara shouted, "No, just get the kit. I won't be able to breathe. Hurry Bret, in the thigh! In the thigh! I don't want to die."

"I'll do it honey. Hang on." He ran over to the backpack, unzipped the side pouch and grabbed the cellular phone and a pamphlet which had the telephone number to the nearby stables. He then unzipped the other portion of the backpack, tossed out some clothes and found the metal box he needed.

"I got it! I got it!" He raced back and knelt down, expecting Clara to respond. But at that moment, lying on the ground, she gasped again for air, clutched her throat, and pleaded with her eyes for Bret to save her. Then suddenly her eyes closed. She became unconscious and lifeless like a cold corpse. Clara's face and extremities exhibited marked swelling. Cyanosis of the lips began to set in.

Bret frantically unclasped the first aid kit and flung it open. He glanced at everything, then picked up a syringe wrapped in cellophane. He tore off the wrapper, looked toward the sky and said, "Please God, please, help me save her. He quickly tore the cap from the syringe and jabbed the needle directly into Clara's right thigh. Although the sharp needle had released the Epinephrine into her system, she remained silent and motionless for a few more minutes. Bret checked for a pulse and began respirations, hoping that as soon as the drug kicked in, the airway would open up.

Believe me, I've worked in the field long enough to know that she was a goner without that injection. Deadly chaos had broken loose inside her. War is such a horror, even for someone who has fought thousands of battles.

Her blood thickened, fluid filled her lungs. I raced over to her heart, and sure enough, it was slowing down and she was on the verge of convulsions due to the lack of blood and oxygen to her brain.

Ige troops had activated the enzymes, then the mast cell granules began to over-react to the bee's venom by releasing histamine and other biochemical warfare. Of course, all of my buddies were doing their jobs. Antibodies make very conscientious soldiers. Like I said, it was impossible to get through to many of them and change their thinking. They were trained, conditioned to react a certain way, but the good that evolved from this unfortunate incident is the fact that I did manage to pull, like I said, some fellow comrades out of the darkness, and even, believe it or not, those two antigens.

They finally figured it out; how we can be so destructive ourselves, rather than preserving and protecting and even to the point of fatal over-reactions. It never made any sense in this line of work. Try to counter-attack and do some good, and look what can happen. I figure it's all a matter of balance, finding that immunological equilibrium.

I handed them all my sob story about Marin, how we lost her. That's what did it, and the close call with Clara. Then I played the Army scout, made sure the Granules did their job, but then proceeded to beg them all to help me prevent the fatal reaction. You see, we are the good guys, but the sad truth is that we can be as dangerous as we are helpful. The antigen troops are the bad guys, the relentless antagonists, but there are ways to fight them and win.

Clara won, thanks to an antidote that was on hand and administered properly, and a follow-up emergency rescue. Every time I hear a helicopter whirling by in the air these days, I think of that huge yellow and orange monster of a chopper that descended from the clear blue and transported Clara on what certainly could have been a "flight for life".

The shot stabilized her, but who knows if she was out of the woods yet. That close to death and you don't want to take any chances. Bret was lucky he could get through to the horse stable so they could call 911 and dispatch the hospital helicopter. The medics got as close as they could to us. That was another problem, transporting, by foot, Clara on the spine board to the helicopter location. I can still hear the sound of the engines and the chopper blades swirling around on take off and the pilot shouting, "Air Rescue One to dispatcher, we're in the air now and have the stable post-anaphylactic patient on board."

I noticed the dedicated look in the flight nurse's face as she adjusted the liter valve on the oxygen. What a close call, I thought to myself. I'm getting too old for this kind of adventure.

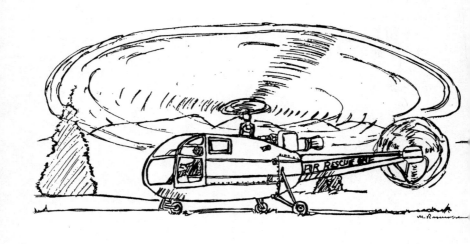

CHAPTER 18

So that's it. That's my story, and I suppose if you're an antibody, or if anyone in your family, yourself, or your friends have ever had any experiences with allergies or asthma, or maybe if you study this stuff or if you work in the field, you'll find it interesting. If not, that's your choice. All I know is, it's not my problem any more. I've done my job, and what I felt I had to do. After all, who else could have told you the inside story?

George and I are checking on some sources, see if we can get transferred to some controlled, mild case down south near the beaches or something. And it's going to be with someone who wears one of those bracelets and carries an emergency kit, just in case. We're getting too old for this kind of drama in our lives. Clara knows how to take care of herself, and some specialist troops took over since a bunch of the others were wiped out, so she'll be fine.

It's time for me to take some time out for living, not in fear, not in frustration, not in anger or pain, not misunderstood, not playing "hero", and certainly not chained to the past. One other thing that George and I found comfort in during our ordeal with the ones we lost, or others who encountered very close brushes with death, was the ability to accept the fact that sometimes an antibody does what he/she has to do, not what he/she wants to do. It took us both a long time to learn that. You know what I'd like though, most of all? To be myself. I just want to be Henry, all masks and pretensions removed.

I feel whole again, and free, really free. At last. Although a clergybody once told me that, "In actuality, commitment is the truest kind of freedom". Maybe I'll feel like an old goatbody out to pasture. The field of allergy and immunology is all I really know. But I also know, within my heart, that it's time to let go.

One final thought. If I had the chance to tell allergic victims one thing, I'd tell them that bodies, minds, and spirits that try hard to heal themselves, against all odds, no matter how sick, disillusioned, or handicapped, no matter how long it might take, they're the real heroes. A poet, Kay Kaye, once wrote, "Survivors are among us, from concentration camps, from tragedies, from sickness, from the dungeons of neglect and abuse. But only for a short time in their lives were they 'Victims,' because from very early on, they began surviving or else they wouldn't still be here."

What it comes down to in the final analysis is that nobody can bring you peace but yourself. I'd try to convince hypersensitive individuals to exercise an indomitable will and personal responsibility, as much as possible, so that they wouldn't have to feel helpless or hopeless, or overwhelmed by threatening external conditions. The body's state of immunity and equilibrium will continuously be challenged throughout a sufferer's lifetime.

However, the individual's state of mind and willingness to learn about and work toward the possibilities for better health will play such an important part in determining his or her quality of life.

Like Frankl, one of the human heroes I've read about, he could not and did not deny the concentration camp's existence and suffering which he endured. But, he did manage to rely on his most self-transcendent capabilities to deny the limitations of a specific detrimental environment and set of circumstances. Nothing, absolutely nothing, could take away or destroy his will to live and right to enjoy life, and hope and dream for a happier, healthier, freer tomorrow. Same thing with the survivors I've been reading about in the paper lately, some innocent people sitting in prisons who, according to actual facts and evidence, have proven their innocence. But it seems, nobody will listen. I can't imagine whole families, years destroyed, because of actual crimes or some distortion of justice. And yet they survive, just like Frankl, somehow.

Finally, in regards to my fellow antibodies and the allergic/asthmatic population, I'd wish them all good luck. "The best of luck to you," from Henry. I conveyed the same sentiments to my buddy George one day..

"Say, Henry, tell them I said good luck too."

"Folks, George wishes everyone good luck too."

"You know Henry, the boss just handed me a scoop about a case out west, in California, lots of sunshine and sandy beaches, just what we wanted."

"Well, what are we waiting for?" I asked excitedly.

"Okay, let's go. There is one thing though. It seems we've been promoted to research, for the big one, AIDS. Now don't get touchy, let me expla...."

But George didn't get the chance to finish. He knew by the look on my face that I didn't want any part of it.

"Oh no you don't," I frowned and shook my head fervently. "There are two diseases that I flatly refuse to work on. You know how I feel about AIDS and cancer. Allergies and asthma are discouraging enough sometimes."

I knew progress was being made in the two fields, but cancer hit close to home, too many relatives or favorite people lost to it, and AIDS, all I could remember were the years I spent with Ryan, a young kid who eventually lost his brave battle. He was a real trooper. All I said was, "Sure George, remember Ryan, all those years of fighting, then we lost him. I'm not going through that again."

My dazed expression must have been apparent to him.

"Henry, Henry! Are you listening?" He shouted. "This is different, Henry, believe me. We'll be working with some specialists, MABS (monoclonal antibodies). Immunotherapy is finally recognized as a crucial modality. They're listening to us Henry, understand?"

"Mono what?' I backtracked.

"Oh let me explain it to you later. Just say you'll think about it," George pleaded. "We're a team pal. I need you. We can do some good."

After a few moments of serious contemplation, all of my mental barriers to George's suggestions dissipated. Actually, I felt kind of relieved, to tell you the truth. It's a strange thing about living, seems to be much more worthwhile and exciting when there's purpose and direction involved. "How old did you say this case was?" I asked.

"Only 27, and you know there's a lot of hope at that age, especially with all of this new research, and of course all of our experience, and this lady, I promise, she's a fighter Henry," he rambled on eagerly. "There's even a researcher in St. Louis, Henry, who's stirring up lots of hope, but controversy too. You won't believe this one, but Doctor Homin thinks there's a NON-allergic aspect that's initially responsible for triggering the chain reaction. By preventing the initial reaction early on, within the airway cells, guess what. No asthma. There coming up with all kinds of new, exciting things to try. I'm telling you buddy, it's a good thing we're both on our way to retirement, because, just like that other doctor in Chicago, trying to wipe out all of the IGE battalions, we might be on our way out, as far as the field of allergy and asthma goes."

Here we go again, I thought. Yes indeed, allergy and immunology will lead humankind to many answers and much healing someday, if they'll just listen.

"Yes, indeed, it sure will. Allergies and..."

"It sure will what? What Clara, what are you mumbling about?" Bret loudly requested an answer while he shook Clara's right arm.

"Hmm? What? No. No. Leave me alone. I wanna sleep some more. I don't want to leave this dream yet." Clara rolled over, ignoring her inquisitive husband.

"What dream Clara?" What sure will? What about allergies?" he persisted.

Clara rubbed her eyes, rolled back on her left side, faced Bret and explained in a short cut manner. "It's a long, incredible story honey. I'll tell you all about it later, okay? Right now, I'm tired and I want to sleep in. It was all about this little character, Henry. He was, I mean I guess I was, an antibody inside people's bodies, you know, like Fantastic Voyage. God, I remember all this fighting between the allergies and us, the antibodies. It was awful."

"You've been reading too much of that book, *The Body is the Hero*. Who is that by? Glasser?" He expected an answer.

"Yeah. Yes, Glasser. Hey, by the way, thanks for saving my life last night. You saved me. We were hiking, just like we did last weekend, but this time I got stung by that yellow jacket we saw, then went into anaphylactic shock, and you and the Flight for Life nurse and paramedic rescued me. That was the weird part. One minute I felt like myself, but then, well you know how dreams jump around and don't make sense all the time, all of a sudden, I'd become Henry and I was inside of my body fighting the antigens, literally fighting them with my friend George. He was another antibody. Oh shoot, George isn't real, darn, I'm going to miss him."

"You're right, go back to sleep."

"But I'm awake now. So you get to listen to the whole story. You see, it all started with this girl Marin..."

"Oh no you don't," Bret jumped out of bed. "Not without my coffee."

"All right, all right. But hurry back. Henry and I will be waiting for you."

Two cups of coffee later, Bret returned as promised.

"Okay honey, I'm raring to go now. I want to hear more about your night job of being an antibody. What was his name, Henry?"

"Yeah, Henry. I was Henry and I had a friend, George. He sounded just like Walter Matthau when he talked or laughed. We were soldiers and detectives. I kept talking about all the different cases I'd worked on, allergic and asthmatic victims, like at the clinic. Most lived, but some of them died. I guess I felt guilty about this one girl named Marin that my friends and I had killed, because of an antigen-antibody war. So I must have been telling the story from Henry's perspective and it seemed so real."

"Hmm. Well I'm curious, what's an antibody look like?"

"Well, seemed like I was shaped like the letter Y and, oh yeah, it was funny. We both had on these blue tennis shoes and George had bigger feet than I did."

"I cannot picture you shaped like a Y with blue tennies. Hey, wait a minute. I just read something the other day about antibodies. You say you kept going from case to case. Were these guys old or young, I mean you and George? Because, as you probably know, antibodies don't live a long time and it said something about when the host dies so does the antibody." He said it smartly, as if he had just been promoted to genius. "So there you go, major flaw in you dream. Henry or you couldn't have gone from case to case because if that girl died, then..."

"I cannot absolutely believe this! I'm telling you that I experienced the most incredibly vivid, cartoon-like, yet realistic fantastic voyage through human bodies last night, actually watched and felt what it was like to witness an all out war between antigens and antibodies and you sit here talking about medical correctness. That's like talking syntax to Thoreau or Mark Twain. IT WAS A DREAM DEAR. Remember? Anything can happen in a dream. It doesn't have to make perfect sense. Don't ever go absolutely practical on me, okay? I couldn't stand it."

Bret joked around, puckered his bottom lip and pretended to hold his head down in shame. "Sorry."

" Forgiven. Now let me tell you the rest of the story.
Just try to pretend you're a kid or something. Dispense
with the grown-up critiquing, just for an hour or so."

"Got it, understood. Go for it Clara. Tell me all
about your adventure." He put his arm around her and she
started again, from the beginning.

"Well, like I said, there was this girl, Marin...."

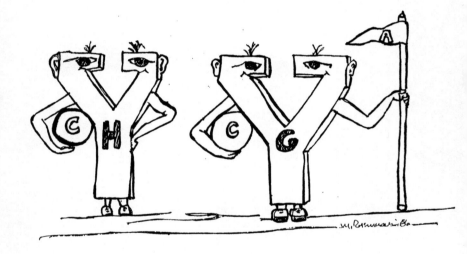